The Midwives' Guide to Key Medical Conditions

For Churchill Livingstone

Commissioning Editor: Mairi McCubbin
Development Editor: Janice Urquhart
Project Manager: Emma Riley
Designer: Charlotte Murray
Illustrator: Ian Ramsden
Illustrations Manager: Gillian Richards

The Midwives' Guide to Key Medical Conditions

PREGNANCY AND CHILDBIRTH

Linda Wylie BA MN RGN RM RMT

Lecturer, School of Health, Nursing and Midwifery, University of Paisley, Scotland, UK

Helen Bryce BSc RN RM ADM MTD

Lecturer, School of Health, Nursing and Midwifery, University of Paisley, Scotland, UK

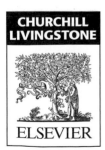

CHURCHILL LIVINGSTONE

ELSEVIER

EDINBURGH   LONDON   NEW YORK   OXFORD   PHILADELPHIA   ST LOUIS   SYDNEY   TORONTO 2008

CHURCHILL
LIVINGSTONE
ELSEVIER

First published 2008
  Reprinted 2008

ISBN: 978-0-443-10387-2

British Library Cataloguing in Publication Data
A catalogue record for this book is available from the British Library

Library of Congress Cataloging in Publication Data
A catalog record for this book is available from the Library of Congress

Notice
Knowledge and best practice in this field are constantly changing. As new research and experience broaden our knowledge, changes in practice, treatment and drug therapy may become necessary or appropriate. Readers are advised to check the most current information provided (i) on procedures featured or (ii) by the manufacturer of each product to be administered, to verify the recommended dose or formula, the method and duration of administration, and contraindications. It is the responsibility of the practitioner, relying on their own experience and knowledge of the patient, to make diagnoses, to determine dosages and the best treatment for each individual patient, and to take all appropriate safety precautions. To the fullest extent of the law, neither the Publisher nor the Authors assume any liability for any injury and/or damage to persons or property arising out of or related to any use of the material contained in this book.

The Publisher

Printed in China

Contents

Preface

The role of the midwife is expanding as new technologies and expectations increase in complexity. The midwife is the expert in normal childbirth, but as the lead professional in the majority of pregnancies and births, must be able to recognize any deviation from the norm and refer her client on to the relevant practitioner. Women with medical disorders that range from the normally mild disease process such as asthma to women with serious complications such as heart lesions are increasing in the pregnant population. Midwives therefore must be able to recognize normal physiology and the early onset of complications.

Most student midwives in the UK go directly into midwifery education at the present time and do not have previous experience as a nurse. There is therefore a need to educate student midwives to understand and recognize medical disorders and pregnancy complications. At present there is no one textbook that revises normal anatomy and physiology, introduces the common medical disorders seen in the woman of childbearing age and identifies the effect these disease processes have on the process of birth. This book is therefore intended to fill this gap.

As with the previous book, *Essential Anatomy and Physiology in Maternity Care*, the references in this book have a dual role. They are intended to identify the source of the information but they are also designed to direct student midwives to good articles, readily accessible, which will give them more in-depth information.

Paisley, 2007

Linda Wylie
Helen Bryce

Acknowledgements

This book would not have been written without the input of my good friend and colleague Helen, who is the co-author of this book. Helen has contributed to all chapters but is also solely responsible for the chapters on the role of the midwife, diabetes, thyroid disorders and anaemia and the haemoglobinopathies.

Other professional colleagues have also been very supportive and we wish to identify Santha in particular for her advice on the care of the neonate; to our fellow lecturers on the midwifery team and of course to all the students who have not been slow in their suggestions for a successful book!

We would also like to thank our families for their patience as we disappeared once again into the computer.

Linda Wylie

Chapter 1

The midwife's role

INTRODUCTION

The formal definition of a midwife was first adopted by the International Confederation of Midwives (ICM) and the International Federation of Gynaecology and Obstetrics (FIGO) in 1972 and 1973, respectively. It was later adopted by the World Health Organization (WHO). The definition was amended by the ICM in 1990 and this amendment was then ratified by the FIGO and the WHO in 1991 and 1992, respectively:

> *A midwife is a person who, having been regularly admitted to a midwifery educational programme, duly recognised in the country in which it is located, has successfully completed the prescribed course of studies in midwifery and has acquired the requisite qualifications to be registered and/or legally licensed to practise midwifery.*
>
> *She must be able to give the necessary supervision, care and advice to women during pregnancy, labour and the postpartum period, to conduct deliveries on her own responsibility and to care for the newborn and the infant. This care includes preventative measures, the detection of abnormal conditions in mother and child, the procurement of medical assistance and the execution of emergency measures in the absence of medical help. She has an important task in health counselling and education, not only for the women, but also within the family and the community. The work should involve antenatal*

education and preparation for parenthood, and extends to certain areas of gynaecology, family planning and child care. She may practise in hospitals, clinics, health units, domiciliary conditions or in any other service

The Association of Radical Midwives states:

A midwife is a specialist who is qualified to give total care to a woman and her baby during pregnancy, labour and after the baby is born. The midwife does not have to call in a doctor unless there is a potential or actual problem which requires medical assistance

(Association of Radical Midwives 2006)

The Royal College of Midwives (RCM) position paper 26: refocusing the role of the midwife states:

Currently, there are a number of developments, both external and internal to the profession that are creating change in midwives' roles and working practices. These changes are not uniform across geography or practice settings. However, they have the potential to challenge midwives' traditional working practices across the UK

(RCM 2006)

Midwives today are facing a dichotomy: at one end of the spectrum, they are constantly being asked to expand their role to incorporate new challenges, new ways of working, new screening programmes and develop new skills, and at the other end midwifery skills are being farmed out to support workers or nurses. It is inconceivable that midwives can be all things to all people, but embarking on change must be carefully thought out, measuring and weighing current practice and ensuring safety and quality to women in our care.

The role of the midwife, from whichever perspective, is diverse and encourages informed decision-making, working in partnership with other health and social care services in a wide variety of care settings, including low and high risk settings and working independently outside the NHS.

Many women have complications or underlying medical conditions that require specialist obstetric and multidisciplinary care during childbearing and midwives also play a pivotal part in this process, delivering the necessary care, providing continuity and support and linking directly or indirectly with all other members of the multidisciplinary team. Basic knowledge and understanding of medical conditions affecting pregnancy and childbearing is only a starting point for today's professional midwife. The midwife has been educated to have a thorough knowledge and understanding of normal childbearing and this is her field of expertise. However, the midwife's knowledge cannot be restricted, as this would be naive and unrealistic but her knowledge and understanding of complications and medical conditions of pregnancy should be slanted towards midwifery care. This is not less than medical care, just different.

There is still a hierarchical element within the National Health Service (NHS), and obstetricians are assumed to have final control. However, midwives must be prepared to be assertive and act as advocates for women when required. It is possible to develop a professional relationship with medical staff where there is mutual trust, and where each member of a team works harmoniously, benefiting from each others' expertise. Midwives need to feel safe and valued as members of the team and management has to reverse the prevailing culture of fragmentation and put in place measures which empower midwives (Curtis et al 2006).

One of the most important attributes of a midwife is competence. Attaining competence is hard work; it requires effort, commitment, responsibility, preparation and above all motivation. Knowledge and understanding of conditions, their management and development of clinical skills leads to competence and fitness for purpose. Fitness for purpose demonstrates the ability and proficiency for practice. Women today require a professionally competent midwife, one who goes that extra step to learn, to hone a skill, or to communicate effectively. Clinical competence is only one facet of care.

Midwives who succeed in professional practice reflect on their care and fully embrace the concept of lifelong learning. They demonstrate qualities of empathy, enthusiasm and assertiveness in all aspects of care. They are professionally supportive of women and colleagues. This is of fundamental importance as all too often, midwives have shirked the professional responsibility of supporting their colleagues in both clinical and management roles, and nowhere is this more important than when caring for women with complications or medical conditions in pregnancy. Critical thinking and reflection in and on practice by every midwife is necessary to raise and maintain standards. Updating knowledge and understanding of specific conditions can be achieved through reading relevant articles, informal discussions, tutorials or fire drills during quiet periods.

Midwifery practice is governed by the Midwives Rules and Standards (NMC 2004b). These rules and standards are designed to protect the public, and also describe the standard one would reasonably expect from someone who is practicing as a midwife or is responsible for the statutory supervision of midwives. Midwives should be familiar with all parts of the rules and standards as they allude to, and define the parameters for safe everyday practice.

In caring for women with 'high risk' pregnancies, the midwife should pay particular attention to the following:

> Rule 6 ...
> 2. Except in emergency, a practising midwife shall not provide any care, or undertake any treatment, which she has not been trained to give.
> 3. In an emergency, or where a deviation from the norm which is outside her current sphere of practice becomes apparent in a woman or baby during the antenatal, intranatal or postnatal periods, a practising midwife shall call such qualified health professional as may reasonably be expected to have the necessary skills and experience to assist her in the provision of care

In essence, this means each midwife is required to personally ensure she develops the requisite skills in order to care for women within her particular sphere of employment. Employers have a responsibility to make provision to enable midwives to develop such skills. This also includes the administration of medicines. In an emergency, a midwife must call on any relevant person to aid her in care, for example a more experienced midwife, a doctor/obstetrician, anaesthetist or paramedic. The midwife is also required to call for medical aid where there is a deviation from normal circumstances.

If when requesting medical aid a doctor either fails to attend, or does not take appropriate action,

this does not relieve the midwife of the responsibility to the woman or infant in her care. The midwife should contact another more senior member of staff and her supervisor of midwives.

In circumstances such as the above, it is essential that the midwife records the time of making a request for medical aid, and documents the time and the reason for the request in both midwifery and medical notes. In law, courts consider that if something alleged to be carried out is not documented, then it was not done.

The Nursing and Midwifery Council considers that record-keeping is fundamental to midwifery practice and helps safeguard the public by promoting high standards of care, communication of information, and an accurate record of care provided, enabling the identification of problems at an early stage (NMC 2005).

Good record-keeping also protects the midwife. If the midwife follows the guidance for record-keeping and documents factually, consistently and accurately as soon as possible following an event and where possible, written with the involvement of the woman concerned, and without abbreviations, jargon or alterations, then the midwife is demonstrating evidence of the care delivered.

It is in the midwife's best interests to maintain good records. It enables her to logically and sequentially document the planning, implementation and evaluation of care, which will aid her to recall events accurately during reports or handovers to midwives or members of the multidisciplinary team and allow others to follow care even in her absence. In addition, logical, sequential and factually accurate recording of information can go far to increase the recognition of the midwife as a legitimate professional.

In order to provide a high standard of care, the midwife must scrutinize her practice to ensure that the care provided is not carried out routinely by habit or tradition, but as result of critically examining current research to identify the best available, current, valid and relevant evidence in order to provide evidence-based practice. This is important in caring for any woman, as well as when caring for women with problems or complications of childbearing, as in this situation, the woman's health may already be compromised and substandard care could further undermine her health.

Supervision of midwives is provided to promote a safe standard of midwifery practice, in order to protect women and babies through a system of support and guidance for every practising midwife in the UK. Individual midwives who are eligible to become supervisors have to undergo a period of preparation. They have a wide remit and are involved in promoting best practice, preventing poor practice and intervening in unacceptable practice. One facet of their roles is to monitor practice through audit and ensuring midwifery practice and decision-making is evidence-based (NMC 2006). Additionally, they are available as experienced professionals to advise and support midwives in gaining the experience they require to care for those women who come into pregnancy with a pre-existing medical condition.

PRECONCEPTION CARE

A total of 5% of babies are born with a defect, which can range from a minor blemish such as a birthmark (although this may not seem minor to the mother and baby), to life-threatening abnormalities of major organs, such as the heart. Some of these defects could be avoided, or the effect reduced, by the mother embarking on a healthy lifestyle well before conception.

Preconception health promotion

Preconception health promotion should be directed towards all women with or without known health risks. It can be delivered by all members of the multidisciplinary team to both partners, in an attempt to achieve optimal health 3–6 months before possible conception. Healthy lifestyle choices are discussed and delivered as part of a school curriculum in parts of the UK.

Issues addressed at a preconception clinic include nutrition and weight, the use of alcohol and tobacco, prescribed and over-the-counter medications and illicit drugs. Environmental issues and hazards should also be considered. The risk of infection, immunizations and pre-existing disease, genetic risks and family planning are all considered. Other areas to consider include domestic violence and infertility.

The midwife can be a vital contributor in offering preconception care. Advertising in the community and providing opportunity during regular antenatal clinics will encourage women to prevail themselves of such a service.

PRENATAL CARE

The booking visit, or the first visit of a pregnant woman with the midwife, is generally considered to be the most significant visit the woman will make during her pregnancy. It can set the scene, if handled sensitively and professionally, for the initiation of a trusting relationship, where midwife and woman become partners in care. It is also an opportunity to assess risk. The booking visit should be carried out in an informal and uninterrupted environment. Privacy is essential, and sufficient time must be allocated to allow the midwife to make enquiries about a range of issues including the woman's family, social, menstrual, medical and obstetrical history. As the interview proceeds, the midwife will be able to conclude when it becomes appropriate to ask more sensitive and personal questions, dealing with areas such as possible domestic abuse.

The midwife will also be able to advise the woman and her family on a healthy pregnancy, covering such topics as nutrition, exercise, medications and other lifestyle issues, and any subjects of concern raised by the woman herself.

There is ongoing debate regarding the frequency of prenatal visits, with many members of the multidisciplinary team suggesting the traditional pattern of visits is unnecessary. The National Institute for Clinical Excellence (NICE) guidelines for antenatal care consider that reducing the number of prenatal visits would give the midwife time to provide individual information and support (NICE 2003).

Having undertaken a thorough medical history from the woman, and taking into consideration any risk factors that have been identified, the midwife and the woman can formulate a plan of care tailored to the individual woman's needs. This should include contact telephone numbers and midwifery notes. Information and contents of the midwifery notes must be discussed with the woman to ensure she fully understands what has been written, and should follow the NMC's guidelines for records and record-keeping (NMC 2005). Part of this process will be to refer the woman on to relevant members of the multidisciplinary team as required (NICE 2003).

The majority of pregnant women are healthy and care can be provided solely by a midwife. However, women with pre-existing disease in pregnancy or other such risk factors should be encouraged to attend a clinic at which all the relevant members of the multidisciplinary team are available. For example, a woman with type 1 diabetes mellitus will require regular consultations with the midwife, obstetrician, diabetologist, dietician, diabetic nurse and other personnel.

A vital function of the booking visit, which has already been briefly alluded to, is the development of a rapport by the midwife with the woman. Ideally, midwifery patterns of care will be constructed to ensure the woman is seen by the same midwife throughout her pregnancy, or, if this is not possible, a minimum number of midwives. Research shows that women prefer a familiar midwife throughout pregnancy and postnatally (DOH 1993). Women prefer continuity of care throughout pregnancy and care should be supplied by a small group of carers in line with NICE guidelines on antenatal care (NICE 2003).

Subsequent prenatal visits should be arranged to suit both woman and midwife. The essence of care at all prenatal visits is to assess the needs of the pregnant woman and outline the principles of care. This care alters and evolves as the pregnancy proceeds and must be reassessed at each subsequent visit but should include the following:

- Clinical observations are taken to establish a baseline for future reference; these include measuring and recording blood pressure, pulse and weight and urinalysis

- An abdominal examination is undertaken to assess maternal and fetal well-being; this may also be supplemented by an ultrasonography, assessing growth and gestational age

- Maternal well-being is also estimated by spending time discussing issues of lifestyle and providing psychological and emotional support

- Screening tests will be offered with a fully balanced explanation, both verbal and written, of their purpose and possible outcomes, at a sufficiently early date to enable the woman to make an informed decision

- Education regarding issues relating to the pregnancy, for example, nutritional supplements, environmental hazards, exercise and benefits should be provided. Place of birth and preparation of a birth plan must also be addressed and all related to the individual woman's wishes. Cultural differences, language barriers and disabilities must also be negotiated for relevant care.

The importance of unbiased, balanced and evidence-based advice cannot be overemphasized, and this, coupled with sufficient time, open-ended dialogue and an unhurried approach, can go a long way to provide client satisfaction.

Using an individualized approach will enable the midwife to choose a time and place for further visits that factor in aspects of childcare, or the need for an interpreter or financial issues. By taking this approach, a woman is more likely to continue with her prenatal visits. The recent Confidential Enquiry into Maternal and Child Health (Lewis & Drife 2004) identified that the women most at risk were those that were most unlikely to attend for prenatal care. The midwife should also take action when she recognizes that a client is not attending for prenatal care and try to make alternative arrangements, such as an evening appointment or a home visit.

Pre-existing conditions, which prior to pregnancy were well controlled, can become unstable and unpredictable. This can cause considerable anxiety for the woman, who may have to endure increased medical appointments and possible childcare problems with possible financial loss. This can be further exacerbated if hospital admission is necessary, and in addition to supportive care, the midwife should facilitate referral to other appropriate agencies (NMC 2004a).

INTRANATAL CARE

All women should be offered the full range of options for place of birth, although women with complications, or pre-existing medical conditions should receive unbiased evidence-based information on which alternatives would benefit her best, with justification as to why this is right for her individual circumstances. Green et al (2000) found that women felt that a known carer was of low priority during labour. What was important was a competent, professionally kind carer who inspired trust.

Women with pre-existing disease or medical complications may find that these existing problems impinge on the labour, leading to more interventions, surveillance and consequently worry and anxiety for the woman. Labour may be viewed as an ordeal to be overcome with the woman having little or no control of the outcome. It is the midwife's responsibility to ensure that the woman is kept fully informed about the plan of care and all likely outcomes so she can prepare herself for these events. If a woman has already experienced medical intervention because of a pre-existing condition, she may be more likely to adapt to obstetric and medical control during her labour.

If a situation arises during late pregnancy or in labour, the woman may have little time to adjust to this and the expected labour and birth experience may not materialize. The woman may then feel disappointed and frustrated. The midwife must be able to support the woman, provide a high standard of clinical care and act as liaison between members of the multidisciplinary team:

In high risk situations the woman's voice can get lost, and the midwife may have to step in and act as advocate where necessary.

Interventions and other procedures can de-personalize labour and it may take all of the midwife's ingenuity to remain sensitive to the emotional care the woman requires. Communication is of utmost importance, providing information and explanation when required, but also knowing when to be quiet and enable the woman to draw on her own intuitive reserves. Learning the act of masterly inactivity is a skill all midwives should cultivate. It involves developing confidence in the woman's ability to labour independently and labour is likely to be more comfortable and

progress more quickly if the woman is in quiet, peaceful private surroundings (Robertson 1997).

The judicious use of touch to relieve backache through massage or using hot towels may be beneficial. Likewise, sips of water or ice can moisten the mouth if the woman is using breathing techniques during contractions. Distraction therapy, such as music can also be beneficial. Analgesia should be administered when required, depending on availability and choice. Epidural anaesthesia is mostly available in obstetric units, but it must be made clear that it restricts the movement of the woman. Women who give birth in an upright position are said to have less pain, less perineal trauma and fewer episiotomies (Ragnar et al 2006).

Caring for women with high risk pregnancy or pre-existing medical conditions can be an anxious time for the inexperienced or newly qualified midwife and where possible, she should work with a more experienced midwife when delivering care. If this is not possible, the midwife must inform the midwife coordinator, as she must not undertake any procedures or treatments that she has not been trained to perform (NMC 2004b).

In addition to the national guidelines produced by NICE or SIGN, protocols and local guidelines can be developed by the multidisciplinary team to provide evidence-based care for many specific medical conditions complicating pregnancy.

Labours are very individual, and women progress better in a warm friendly atmosphere (Robertson 1997). Providing the woman's condition permits her to move freely, during early labour she is better to remain upright as gravity aids progression. Where continuous monitoring or other intervention is necessary, the midwife has to adapt care to accommodate and work around these obstacles, as in many instances, the woman lying in bed is more accommodating for the midwife. Monitoring can be carried out standing or on a chair (a recliner is ideal) – wherever it is carried out, the woman must be comfortable and be the focus of care. Attempting to create an atmosphere of normality should be weighed up between the severity of the woman's condition, local provision of care, and the woman's concept of the ideal birth (Lindsay 2006).

Observations should be as unobtrusive as possible, but should be recorded meticulously in the partograms and midwifery notes so that progress can be evaluated. The woman's views and any discussions regarding her care must also be documented. In addition, obstetrical or medical instructions for care should be evidence-based and similarly, must also be documented. Where emergency situations arise, a second midwife should record drugs and treatment given while the original midwife provides care.

Many labours do not progress due to further complications and instrumental or operative delivery may result. Whatever the situation, women must be able to trust midwives to be focussed, competent and to provide the best possible care.

POSTNATAL CARE

The application of postnatal care will depend on the individual woman's condition following birth. If birth has been achieved by operative or instrumental means or the woman has other complications, then initial care is likely to be provided in a high dependency unit. There, close observation and physical care can be provided.

Psychological care, particularly where a woman has undergone emergency surgery can be problematic. Early identification and management of health problems is necessary to reduce the risk of persistent pain, disability or depression. Referral to other agencies and additional support by maternity care assistants, or peer support initiatives may be necessary. The Sure Start Early Years services are proven to be well received.

The National Service Framework (NSF) for children, young people and maternity services (DOH 2004) states that there are more complaints about postnatal care than any other aspect of maternity care. These complaints focus on conflicting advice on infant feeding, poor hygiene and the quality and availability of hospital food.

The NSF suggest that women's needs could be assessed by midwives but their basic care should be supplied by trained support staff, including infant feeding. Certainly in the current environment where there is a shortage of employed midwives, this may be a short-term solution. The UK government states that it wants to improve the uptake of breast-feeding in all areas. Breast-feeding is the right of all babies and there are many individuals and organizations ready and willing to take over this aspect of care from the midwife. This however, must not be allowed to happen; individuals and organizations can be a welcome adjunct to midwifery care, but caring for women willing to breast-feed is a privilege and a fundamental part of midwifery care.

Midwives must be given the means to provide this education to women, where necessary updating knowledge regarding current practice, and must speak with one voice and provide non-conflicting advice for women. Most importantly, they must spend time with women ensuring they are able and confident in their ability to breast-feed. Peer support can be a positive influence in improving maintenance of breast-feeding in women.

Protecting the public is the remit of the Nursing and Midwifery Council, and mothers and babies are a particularly vulnerable group. The NMC and other professional bodies must therefore lobby parliament to ensure midwives have the means and time to fulfil their professional role. Women and the midwives providing care must not be relegated or discriminated against and maternity services cannot be allowed to become a means of placating women through rhetoric in order to gain election votes.

Medical care is seen by the public as an objective scientific discipline. Such a detached dispassionate model of care can only provide a partial fulfilment of needs. Professional midwifery care during childbearing supersedes this impersonal model and provides a type of care that is individual, gentle and compassionate, as well as evidence-based. This type of social care must not be seen as less important than medical care. There is an inherent fear which pervades our society, where to acknowledge feelings and emotions is perceived as shameful or embarrassing, and which is ultimately disempowering. It would be a mistake to view the care the midwife provides as being less important or as an optional accessory. Not only is this care empowering, it is an essential right for women who are the mothers of future generations.

REFERENCES

Association of Radical Midwives (ARM) 2006 What is a midwife? ARM, Oxford

Curtis P, Ball L, Kirkham M 2006 Why do midwives leave. (Not) being the kind of midwife you want to be. British Journal of Midwifery 14(1):27–31

Department of Health 1993 Changing Childbirth, Part 1: Report of the Expert Maternity Group. DOH, London

Department of Health 2004 National Service Framework for children, young people and maternity services. DOH, London

Green J M, Renfrew M J, Curtis P A 2000 Continuity of carer: what matters to women? A review of the evidence. Midwifery 16(3):186–196

Lewis G, Drife J (eds) 2004 Why Mothers Die 2000–2002: The sixth report of the Confidential Enquiries into Maternal Deaths in the United Kingdom. RCOG Press, London

Lindsay P 2006 Creating normality in a high-risk pregnancy. Practising Midwife 9(1):16–19

National Institute for Clinical Excellence 2003 Antenatal care: Routine care for the healthy pregnant woman. Clinical Guideline 6. NICE, London

Nursing and Midwifery Council 2004a Administration of Medicines. NMC, London

Nursing and Midwifery Council 2004b Midwives rules and standards. NMC, London

Nursing and Midwifery Council 2005 Records and record keeping. NMC, London

Nursing and Midwifery Council 2006 Standards for the preparation and practise of supervisors of midwives. NMC, London

Ragnar I, Altmar D, Tyden T, Olssen S E 2006 Comparison of the maternal satisfaction and duration of labour in two delivery positions – a randomized trial. British Journal of Obstetrics and Gynaecology 113(2):165–170

Robertson A 1997 The midwife companion. Ace Graphics, Australia

Royal College of Midwives 2006 Guidance Paper: Position Paper 26: Refocusing the role of the midwife. RCM, London

Chapter 2

Hypertensive disorders

CHAPTER CONTENTS

INTRODUCTION

Hypertension (high blood pressure) is a relatively common disorder in the developed world. It is one of the leading causes of death in mid- to old age. It is also the second leading cause of direct deaths related to the childbearing process. Both in the general population and in pregnancy and childbirth, hypertension can develop with few signs and symptoms and as such has been described as the silent killer.

Two types of hypertensive disorder exist in women of childbearing age – pre-existing hypertension and gestational hypertension. Pre-existing hypertension is usually the less dangerous of the two conditions depending on the severity of the condition, although it does increase the risks of placental insufficiency, abruptio placentae and superimposed pre-eclampsia. Gestational hypertension includes pre-eclampsia and is associated with increased maternal and fetal morbidity and mortality rates. It is vital therefore that the midwife can recognize those most at risk, monitor them regularly and understand their pathophysiology in order to intervene before the mother or fetus is put at risk by complications of the conditions.

RELEVANT ANATOMY AND PHYSIOLOGY

Blood pressure is the force that drives the cardiovascular system. It is the result of the contraction of the heart on blood, forcing it through the blood vessels. The anatomy of the cardiovascular system is shown in Figure 2.1.

The cardiovascular system consists of the heart, blood and blood vessels – the heart pumps blood around the closed system of arteries and veins.

The heart is composed of four chambers separated into a right and left side by a continuous septum. The right atrium receives deoxygenated blood from the body and directs the blood into the right ventricle where it is pumped out by a muscular contraction of the ventricular wall to the lungs. Here the blood is oxygenated and carbon dioxide is removed. The blood then leaves the respiratory system and is returned to the left atrium where it is passed down to the highly

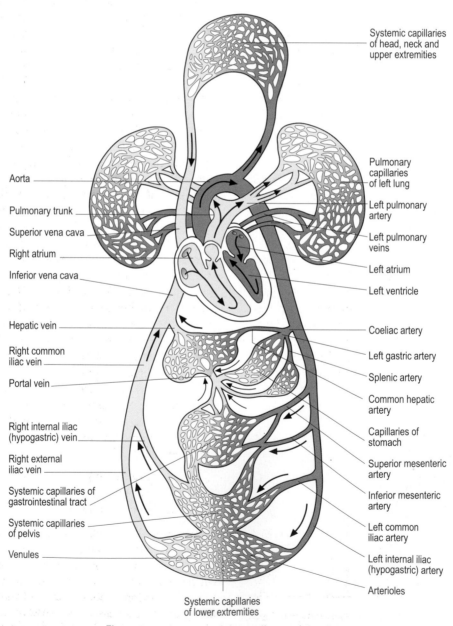

Figure 2.1   Anatomy of the cardiovascular system.

muscular left ventricle. The heart contracts and the blood is moved forcibly out into the largest artery in the body, the aorta, and directed to all parts of the body to transport oxygen, along with other chemicals, to body cells. The pressure of the expulsion of blood from the ventricles on the walls of the blood vessels is the force known as blood pressure. Blood then moves through the circulatory system from the initial area of high pressure to areas of decreasing pressure as shown in Figure 2.2.

In the aorta of a resting healthy young adult, blood pressure rises to about 120 mmHg with each contraction of the ventricles of the heart, the systolic measurement, falling to approximately 80 mmHg (diastole) when the heart is at rest.

Blood pressure is dependent on two factors:

1. Cardiac output
2. Peripheral resistance

Cardiac output is the volume of blood which passes through systemic or pulmonary blood vessels each minute. Cardiac output equals the heart rate multiplied by the stroke volume (amount of blood leaving the heart), i.e. 70 beats × 70 mL, which equals approximately 5 L (litres) of blood.

Should the heart fail to beat efficiently or should there be an insufficient amount of blood in the heart, cardiac output will decrease and blood pressure will decrease also, thus creating hypotension. For example, haemorrhage would cause a decrease in stroke volume and thus ultimately in cardiac output and blood pressure. Body cells will become starved of oxygen, and nutrients

and waste products such as carbon dioxide will accumulate, upsetting the fine acid-base balance required for normal cellular metabolism.

Should cardiac output increase due to increased heart rate or stroke volume or a combination of the two, blood pressure will rise. Increased cardiac output may be required if greater demands are made on the body such as during exercise, with body cells requiring increased amounts of oxygen, glucose and other nutrients. Alternatively, increased cardiac output may be required to push blood through damaged blood vessels, such as in atherosclerosis. This is hypertension.

Peripheral resistance is the extent to which the diameters of blood vessels resist the flow of blood. Resistance in the aorta is very low due to the large diameter of the blood vessel and its proximity to the left ventricle of the heart. Blood pressure at this point is therefore high and blood moves easily through the larger arteries. However, as blood moves into the smaller peripheral arteries, the diameter of these individual vessels decreases, causing a resistance to the flow of blood. Blood pressure begins to fall. This is seen most dramatically in the arterioles, where mean arterial blood pressure (MAP) more than halves – from approximately 85 mmHg to 35 mmHg. By the time blood has passed through the tiny capillaries, MAP has decreased further to about 15 mmHg. Thus, blood pressure in the venous system is very low. The venous blood vessels are anatomically altered to prevent back flow of blood returning to the heart by the presence of valves.

Resistance refers therefore to the opposition to blood flow through the circulatory system as a result of friction of the blood with blood vessel walls. Friction and therefore resistance depends on three factors:

1. Viscosity of the blood
2. Blood vessel length
3. Blood vessel diameter.

Viscosity is the 'thickness' of the blood, i.e. the ratio of blood cells and other solids such as proteins to the fluid part of blood – plasma. In conditions such as dehydration, the blood contains a high proportion of solids, and is less easy to move along the blood vessels. Resistance, due to friction along the vessel walls, will be increased. Where

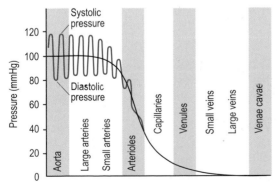

Figure 2.2 Comparison of blood pressure in type of blood vessel.

solids such as red blood cells are decreased, resistance is also decreased.

Blood vessel length affects resistance to blood flow which is directly proportional to the length of a blood vessel; the longer the blood vessel, the higher the resistance.

Blood vessel diameter also affects resistance but is inversely proportional to the diameter of the blood vessel. The narrower the diameter, the more difficult it becomes for blood to move through it. Resistance is increased.

The sum total of all the influences detailed above throughout the circulatory system produces the *total peripheral resistance*. The biggest influence is found in the smallest blood vessels of the body, the arterioles, capillaries and venules. In addition, arteriole walls contain smooth muscle, which can be influenced by chemicals to contract or relax, causing increased diameter, vasodilation, or decreased diameter, vasoconstriction, and thus have the greatest effect on peripheral resistance.

Control of blood pressure

Blood pressure must be maintained at a level sufficient to meet the needs of all the systems and organs of the body. Additionally, local demands on body organs and structures are constantly changing. In order to meet these demands a mechanism must be in place to adjust the blood flow to these areas according to need. For example, when undertaking exercise, the muscles of the limbs require an increase in oxygen and glucose in order to continue functioning. Blood flow is rapidly increased to these areas therefore by relaxation of the smooth muscles in local arteriole walls – vasodilation. Blood flow to the brain however, remains nearly constant.

Blood flow and thus pressure is therefore constantly being adjusted throughout the body centrally via the nervous system, peripherally by hormonal intervention and locally by autoregulation.

Central regulation

Central control is found in the medulla of the brain. Clusters of neurons in the medulla regulate heart rate, force of contraction of the ventricles of the heart (contractility) and blood vessel diameter.

Information is gathered from many sources and sent to this area – the cardiovascular centre – to enable it to adjust the heart's function according to need.

Baroreceptors are found in the walls of arteries and veins and in the right atrium of the heart. These are collections of sensory nerve cells that respond to changes in pressure or stretch. Thus, if these receptors identify an increase in blood pressure they send this information to the cardiovascular centre, which will decrease both heart rate and force of contraction. Alternatively, if a fall in stretch of the blood vessel walls is detected, indicating a fall in blood pressure, this information, when sent to the cardiovascular centre, will result in an increase in heart rate and force and a decrease in blood vessel diameter – vasoconstriction, to increase blood pressure.

Chemoreceptors are situated in the carotid artery and aorta and monitor chemicals in the blood. Chemoreceptors monitor levels of carbon dioxide, pH and oxygen. If there is an increase in carbon dioxide levels or pH, or a decrease in oxygen levels, this information is again sent to the cardiovascular centre in the medulla, and the cardiac rate and rhythm alter accordingly.

The cerebral cortex, limbic system and hypothalamus also play a part in this central control. In response to information received from the body, these organs constantly detect and control other factors that may affect blood pressure such as body temperature (the hypothalamus) and excitement and anticipation, via the cortex and limbic system.

Hormonal regulation

Several hormones are involved in the regulation of blood pressure:

- Adrenaline and noradrenaline from the adrenal cortex increase the rate and force of cardiac contractions, and affect the diameter of blood vessels
- Antidiuretic hormone from the hypothalamus causes vasoconstriction if there is serious loss of blood due to haemorrhage
- The renin–angiotensin pathway increases blood pressure by vasoconstriction and by stimulating the release of aldosterone. Aldosterone

Box 2.1 Juxtaglomerular apparatus

The juxtaglomerular apparatus is the name given to a microscopic region of the nephron in which the afferent arteriole and the final portion of the ascending limb of the loop of Henle come into close proximity. Both of these structures contain specialized cells which control the flow of blood into the nephron and ultimately the blood pressure.

The juxtaglomerular cells situated in the afferent arteriole detect the pressure of the blood contained within the vessel. If blood pressure drops, these cells secrete renin into the bloodstream, which initiates the renin–angiotensin pathway, resulting in vasoconstriction of arterioles conserving an adequate glomerular filtration rate (GFR) and increasing blood pressure throughout the body. In addition, the macula densa, a region of specialized cells in the adjacent renal tubule, measures sodium levels in the filtrate. If sodium levels fall, the macula densa cells stimulate the juxtaglomerular cells to secrete renin.

In addition to vasoconstriction, angiotensin II, which is the final product of the renin–angiotensin pathway, also stimulates the release of antidiuretic hormone to retain fluid and aldosterone to retain sodium in the body.

increases sodium and water reabsorption in the kidneys (Box 2.1)

- Atrial natriuretic peptide is released from cells in the atria of the heart when blood pressure is high, resulting in vasodilation and the loss of salt and water via the kidneys.

Autoregulation

Autoregulation is a local automatic control of blood flow to a specific organ or structure of the body according to its needs. Oxygen levels are the stimulus for autoregulation in most areas of the body, although chemicals such as ions and metabolic products such as lactic acid are the direct cause. If tissues are working hard, available oxygen will be rapidly used up and this will stimulate local arterioles to release such factors causing vasodilation and an increased volume of blood to that area. Although the brain receives a fairly constant supply of blood, blood distribution changes dramatically according to which area is currently most active.

HYPERTENSION IN THE GENERAL POPULATION

It is thought that at least 18% of the UK population suffers from hypertension; the majority, at least 95%, of unknown cause (Beevers et al 2001). Hypertension is present in 1–6% of women of childbearing age (Magee 2001). Hypertension has been termed the 'silent killer' because the sufferer commonly has no symptoms and is only diagnosed through screening or when the disease manifests itself in a complication of the disorder. Hypertension is present in up to 10% of all pregnancies either as a pre-existing disease (5–15% of the total) or as a disorder specific to pregnancy, pre-eclampsia (Lloyd 2003). Diagnosing and treating the hypertensive diseases of pregnancy is very challenging and may involve a balancing act between the health of the mother and the maturity of the fetus.

Aetiology

In the majority of cases, hypertension has no known cause. This is termed primary or essential hypertension. In a small number of cases however, hypertension is secondary to another disease process, such as renal disease, which accounts for one-third of cases, or other disease processes such as adrenal defects as found in phaeochromocytoma or Cushing's syndrome, or as a complication of drug therapy.

Pathophysiology of hypertension

Essential hypertension

Although the exact cause of essential hypertension is not known, it is probable that many interrelated factors contribute to increased blood pressure. Normal blood pressure is dependent on a balance between cardiac output and peripheral resistance as described above. Most people with essential hypertension have a normal cardiac output but a raised peripheral resistance. The reason for this is unclear. Factors that may contribute to this may include a familial tendency, diet, obesity, insulin resistance, fetal development and neurovascular anomalies (Beevers et al 2001). Whatever the cause, the result is an inappropriate decrease in the diameter of the arterioles resulting in increased peripheral resistance. As a result, cardiac rate and/or stroke volume increases to produce a blood pressure sufficient to overcome this resistance and get sufficient blood with gases and nutrients to the cells of the body to enable metabolism to take place.

Secondary hypertension

Secondary hypertension is the result of an identifiable abnormality which causes increased peripheral resistance (Gutierrez & Petersen 2002). For example, renal disease may result in decreased renal perfusion stimulating the kidneys to release increased amounts of renin; an adrenal tumour or hyperthyroidism will stimulate increased amounts of catecholamines. Inappropriately increased levels of renin or catecholamines will cause vasoconstriction and thus increase peripheral resistance. Cardiac output will increase in order to raise blood pressure sufficiently to get sufficient gases and nutrients to all the cells of the body.

Signs and symptoms Hypertension is generally asymptomatic. It is usually diagnosed during routine physical examination when an increased blood pressure is observed, or secondary to another disorder as described above. Diagnosis may result from examination of the eyes by the ophthalmologist in those with visual impairments. Should hypertension be undiagnosed during such examinations, the first evidence may be due to a complication of the condition such as cardiac or renal disease, or stroke.

Those who do experience symptoms complain of vague symptoms such as occipital headache, weakness, dizziness, epistaxis or visual disturbances.

Diagnosis Diagnosis of hypertension is made when resting blood pressures >140 mmHg systolic and/or 90 mmHg diastolic are observed (Box 2.2).

Treatment The goal of successful management of both essential and secondary hypertension is to lower and maintain blood pressure below 140/90 in order to prevent complications or death by permanent damage to sensitive organs of the body such as the heart, brain, kidneys and eyes. Additionally, the patient will be investigated for secondary causes although these will only be present in a minority of cases.

Treatment will depend on the degree of hypertension and the presence of end organ damage. In

---

Box 2.2 White coat hypertension

This is a condition in which patients display an increased blood pressure when in hospital or other clinical environment which is not apparent at home. No signs of stress such as tachycardia are present and thus it is difficult to determine the true blood pressure from a single measurement. White coat hypertension therefore describes a situation in which anxiety increases blood pressure. In the absence of any other indicators of hypertension, the midwife should attempt to develop a good relationship with the woman and her family and reassure her that her anxiety is the likely cause of her rise in blood pressure. She should then arrange to see her, preferably in her own home, to repeat the test.

---

the absence of an underlying pathology, treatment will include lifestyle changes as well as pharmacology if merited. Antihypertensive drug therapy is usually introduced when there is a sustained systolic of 160 mmHg or diastolic of 100 mmHg or more.

Lifestyle changes All patients with hypertension will be advised about lifestyle. For those with mild hypertension, changes in diet, a reduction of stress and a decrease in salt intake may be all that is required to reduce blood pressure to a level that will prevent complications to body organs and tissues. Even in those with a more severe degree of hypertension, lifestyle changes may slow down the development of complications of the condition. Areas in which the patient will be advised and supported to make changes are:

- Diet including weight reduction if necessary, healthy eating, salt reduction, alcohol consumption
- Exercise once the hypertension is under control to help achieve and maintain a satisfactory weight
- Smoking cessation, as smoking confers an additional risk factor in the development of hypertension
- Stress management – although the relationship between stress and hypertension has not been proved, stress reduction and the use of relaxation techniques has been shown to be beneficial to health promotion.

Drug therapy Severe hypertension will be treated pharmacologically in an attempt to prevent further damage to body organs and tissues. The medical practitioner has a range of oral medications that can be used in the treatment of hypertension:

- Vasodilators such as hydralazine, which act predominantly on the smooth muscle of arterioles
- Angiotensin converting enzyme (ACE) inhibitors such as captopril, which reduce peripheral resistance by blocking the conversion of angiotensin I to angiotensin II
- Diuretics such as thiazides and furosemide (frusemide), which reduce interstitial fluid causing vessel wall stiffness. Regular monitoring of serum potassium is essential as hypokalaemia can be a side-effect of these drugs (Kennedy 2002)
- Drugs which act on the central nervous system.
  - Centrally acting drugs, such as methyldopa, which decrease sympathetic nervous system activity
  - Beta blockers, such as propranolol, which block beta receptors in the sympathetic nervous system – these drugs reduce blood pressure but have the added advantage of being cardioprotective – they inhibit the rate and force of cardiac contraction as well as reducing the normal cardiac response to stress and exercise.
  - Alpha blockers, such as prazosin, which result in vasodilation of peripheral arterioles
  - Calcium channel blockers, such as nifedipine, which relax smooth muscle in arterioles.

Prognosis Long-term hypertension is a serious condition resulting in vascular and organ damage. The higher the blood pressure, the higher the risk of complications. Arterial walls become thickened and sclerosed reducing blood supply to tissues. Areas of necrosis may develop which may rupture under pressure. Thrombosis is likely. The most vulnerable organs to damage from sustained hypertension are:

The heart Increased workload results in hypertrophy of the myocardium, and the coronary arteries are unable to supply sufficient blood to this muscle. Angina pectoris or myocardial infarction may result.

The brain Increased pressure in the narrowed and damaged cranial blood vessels may cause rupture or blockage of the vessels and death of brain tissue – a stroke.

The kidneys Renal blood vessels will also become narrowed and weakened with resultant thromboses and dysfunction.

The eyes Retinal capillaries may rupture causing degenerative changes.

HYPERTENSION IN PREGNANCY AND CHILDBIRTH

Overview

Hypertensive disorders occur in up to 10% of all pregnancies and contribute significantly to both maternal and fetal mortality and morbidity rates (Lloyd 2003). Caring for the pregnant women with hypertension is a considerable challenge for the multidisciplinary team. As in the general population, there are seldom any signs or symptoms of hypertension and as the midwife is the primary care giver in the majority of pregnancies, she must be alert for this condition. Screening early in pregnancy will identify women with pre-existing hypertension. Ongoing examination throughout pregnancy will identify women developing pregnancy-induced hypertension or pre-eclampsia. However, hypertension may be a late sign of pre-eclampsia and thus the health of both mother and fetus may be compromised before the condition is detected.

Relevant physiological changes in the cardiovascular system in pregnancy

During pregnancy, the cardiovascular system must meet the increasing demands of both the pregnant woman and the growing fetus. In the heart, cardiac output will increase by up to 40% during the first and second trimesters of pregnancy (Murray 2003). Both stroke volume and heart rate will contribute to this. The raised cardiac output enables blood to flow through the added circulation formed in the enlarging uterus and placental bed, and also to meet the extra needs of other organs of the mother's body.

Blood vessels increase in number and length to supply the placenta. Vasodilation occurs as a result of the action of the hormone progesterone on the smooth muscle of the vessel walls. Plasma volume increases by up to 50% and the number of blood cells by up to 18% during pregnancy to compensate for the apparent loss in blood volume resulting from the presence of extra blood vessels and vasodilation (Blackburn 2002). A resultant lowering of blood pressure in mid-pregnancy may contribute to feelings of lightheadedness and fatigue in the mother. The disproportionate increase in plasma volume over the number of blood cells and proteins present in circulating blood may result in the loss of fluid to the interstitial fluid compartment in the capillary bed, giving rise to generalized oedema in many pregnant women.

Hypertensive diseases of pregnancy

There have been many attempts to classify the hypertensive disorders of pregnancy. However, it has proved difficult to differentiate between one condition and another, as there are many common signs and symptoms. Also, every woman responds differently to the condition as her body attempts to compensate for the pathological changes that are taking place in her organs and systems. Indeed, in some women the complications may occur before the condition has even been diagnosed, e.g. eclampsia may occur in women who have been normotensive throughout pregnancy.

In this book, an attempt will be made initially to define each condition and look at the progress of the disease state. For the purpose of management of the conditions however, a combined approach will be taken in order to consider the response of the woman and the fetus to the condition, whatever its classification.

Classification of hypertensive disorders in pregnancy

For ease of understanding, the hypertensive disorders of pregnancy will be described using the following classification:

- Essential hypertension
- Essential hypertension with superimposed pregnancy-induced hypertension
- Pregnancy-induced hypertension (PIH)
- Pre-eclampsia
- Eclampsia.

Essential hypertension

Approximately 5% of pregnant woman present with hypertension at their first visit to the antenatal clinic (Soydemir & Kenny 2006). Hypertension may have been previously diagnosed or this may be the first time the condition has been identified. Pre-existing hypertension is known as chronic or essential hypertension. The possible causes and treatment of the condition have been discussed earlier in this chapter. In pregnancy, essential hypertension is more common in older, multiparous women and may occur secondary to renal disease or another disease process, such as systemic lupus erythematosus. Commonly used antihypertensives are not known to be teratogenic; however, any antihypertensives should be continued in early pregnancy only if anticipated benefits outweigh potential risks (Magee 2001).

Diagnosis   Essential hypertension may be difficult to diagnose early in pregnancy due to the normal hypotensive changes of early pregnancy. Commonly however, the blood pressure is found to be 140/90 or more, but usually with no oedema or proteinuria. Essential hypertension is not commonly associated with poor mortality or morbidity rates unless it results in placental insufficiency, placental abruption or superimposed PIH or pre-eclampsia (Gilbert & Harmon 1998).

Management of essential hypertension   Management of essential hypertension will depend on the severity of the condition. The intention will be to maintain a blood pressure of <150/100. Investigations may be carried out for damage to other organs associated with hypertension, such as retinopathy, heart disease or renal disease.

Antihypertensives may be indicated to control hypertension. However, as the reason for the increased blood pressure will be to ensure sufficient blood is reaching the tissues and organs of the body, a reduction in blood pressure may cause placental insufficiency. Other areas of management of this condition will include advising rest and a balanced diet, with control of weight gain. Monitoring of fetal growth will be essential with the possible need for early induction if the fetus is considered to be seriously compromised.

Complications of essential hypertension in pregnancy

Essential hypertension with superimposed pregnancy-induced hypertension Superimposed pregnancy-induced hypertension or pre-eclampsia may develop. These are serious complications of essential hypertension, as this indicates that the body is no longer able to adequately compensate for the underlying pathology that is preventing blood delivering gases and nutrients to the tissues and organs of the body. The prognosis in these circumstances is likely to be poor. This will be covered in more depth in the following sections.

Other possible complications are renal failure, a cerebral vascular accident ('stroke') or rarely, encephalopathy.

Pregnancy-induced hypertension

Pregnancy-induced hypertension (PIH) is a condition in which blood pressure increases after the 20th week of pregnancy. Proteinuria is not present. A raised blood pressure before the 20th week is indicative of essential hypertension, as discussed previously.

Causes of pregnancy-induced hypertension The cause of PIH is not known. However, it has been associated with cases where there is an enlarged placenta, such as hydatidiform mole or multiple pregnancy, or in cases where circulation to the placenta may be compromised, such as in diabetes. In most cases however, there is no obvious cause. The incidence of the condition varies with race and location and appears to be more prevalent with increasing age. As there is a rise in blood pressure with no proteinuria, it seems probable that the condition is an indication that the body is no longer able to compensate for circulatory pathology related to essential hypertension with the added vasculature related to the placenta and fetus.

Diagnosis The presence of a diastolic blood pressure of >110 mmHg on any occasion or >90 mmHg on two or more occasions, 4 h apart, is considered to be diagnostic. No proteinuria is present.

Management The woman with PIH needs careful surveillance. An initial assessment will determine whether any complications of the condition are already present. This assessment will consider maternal and fetal condition.

Maternal condition A full physical examination will be carried out to determine the presence of any conditions that may be causing an increase in blood pressure unrelated to the pregnancy. Serial blood pressure measurements will be undertaken over time to give an indication of the severity of the condition. Ultrasound examination will be undertaken to rule out the presence of a molar pregnancy. A blood sample will be obtained for a full blood count, serum urates and urea and electrolytes. Urinalysis will identify the presence of substances not normally found, such as protein and glucose. These tests will also rule out complications such as thrombocytopenia, liver and renal damage.

Fetal condition Abdominal examination will be carried out to determine the growth of the fetus. Ultrasound examination will also consider this. A cardiotocograph will be performed to assess the health of the fetus and will also identify evidence of good fetal movement.

In the absence of any indications of maternal or fetal complications, the woman will be reassessed regularly throughout her remaining weeks of pregnancy.

Management of maternal and/or fetal compromise will be considered later in the chapter as this depends less on the cause and more on maternal and fetal condition.

Pre-eclampsia

Pre-eclampsia and its complications is one of the most serious conditions to affect the pregnant woman and her baby and is responsible for the deaths of three to five women and between 500 and 600 babies in the UK per year (www.apec.org.uk). In the most recent Confidential Enquiries into Maternal and Child Health (CEMACH), 14 deaths were attributed to pre-eclampsia and/or eclampsia; nine women died of intracranial haemorrhage, one from ARDS, two from multi-organ failure and two from disseminated intravascular coagulation (DIC) (Lewis & Drife 2004). Although not fully understood, pre-eclampsia appears to be caused by a defect in the placenta. It is usually symptomless in the early stages and detected during routine antenatal examinations. As midwives are the lead professionals responsible for monitoring the majority of women during pregnancy, it is essential that they can recognize the condition and act appropriately.

Incidence   Approximately 2–3% of all pregnant women will develop pre-eclampsia (RCOG 2006).

Aetiology   Pre-eclampsia has a complex aetiology, which appears to be the result of an interplay between abnormal genetic, immunological and placental factors (Duckett et al 2001). A familial tendency is suggested by the three- to four-fold increase in incidence in first degree relatives of affected women. Nutritional deficiencies have also been considered (Atallah et al 2006, Robinson 2004).

The possibility of an overwhelming immune response to the foreign proteins of the fetus and placenta also has considerable support. This could explain why pre-eclampsia is more common in primigravida women, with women who have changed partners and with those who have used barrier methods of contraception. Length of cohabitation also appears to be a factor (Koelman et al 2000). These women will have had limited exposure to their partners semen and little opportunity to develop the necessary antibodies to the foreign proteins.

The placental factor leads to abnormal placentation during the second wave of trophoblastic invasion at 14–15 weeks' gestation. Normally, the trophoblast disrupts the muscular and elastic walls of the spiral arteries of the decidua – in pre-eclampsia, this does not occur.

Although there is no known direct cause of pre-eclampsia, there appears to be a number of predisposing factors associated with the condition (Milne et al 2005):

- Primigravidous women especially <19 or >40 years
- Primipaternity – first pregnancy with this partner
- ≥10 years since last baby
- Previous history of pre-eclampsia
- Family history of pre-eclampsia (mother or sister)

- Proteinuria at booking
- Booking diastolic blood pressure ≥80 mmHg
- Pre-existing medical conditions, especially diabetes or essential hypertension
- Multiple pregnancy
- BMI ≥35.

Pathophysiology   During the development of the placenta in early pregnancy, the trophoblast burrows deep into the endometrium of the uterus (the decidua) and replaces the musculo-elastic lining of the spiral arteries. This results in large structureless sinuses, which can supply the hugely expanded blood flow required especially in the third trimester (Redman & Sargent 2001). These dilated vessels are no longer influenced by hormones. In pre-eclampsia, adaptation of the spiral arteries by the trophoblast does not occur (Morley 2004). As a result, blood supply to the placenta is limited (Figs 2.3, 2.4). As demand increases during fetal growth, supply is insufficient and the placenta becomes ischaemic.

Placental ischaemia results in the release of substances that are toxic to the maternal body in general and the circulatory system in particular.

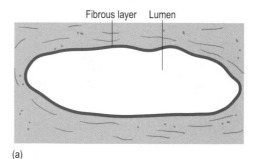

(a)

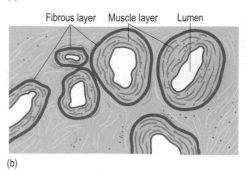

(b)

Figure 2.3   Spiral arteries of the endometrium. (a) Normal structure (NB: Lack of muscle layer). (b) Abnormal structure (NB: Presence of muscle layer).

The endothelial cells of the blood vessels of the body are particularly at risk. These cells are responsible for the integrity of the blood vessel walls. Endothelial cells produce substances, such as prostacyclin and nitric acid, which are responsible for vasodilation in response to circulating hormones. Production of these substances is therefore compromised. Additionally, vasoconstrictors such as thromboxane and lipid peroxides are produced in increased quantities from the damaged endothelial cells. The end-result of this chemical imbalance is a seven-fold increase in the production of thromboxane over prostacyclin and a corresponding increase in vascular sensitivity to angiotensin II. Blood vessels are thus inappropriately constricted in diameter.

These biochemical changes affect the whole of the body. Generalized vasospasm occurs, leading to poor perfusion of blood to the tissues and organs of the body. The degree to which the organs can function under these circumstances results in

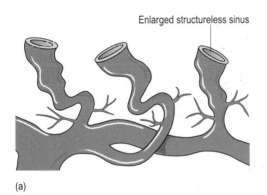

(a)

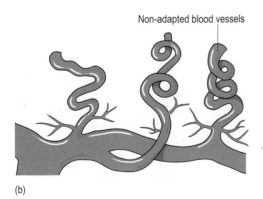

(b)

Figure 2.4 Placental blood supply from spiral arteries. (a) Normal adaptation: dilated blood vessels. (b) Lack of dilation of blood vessels.

varying effects on the woman's body and on fetal condition. Blood pressure rises in the majority of women and increased endothelial cell permeability results in loss of fluid and proteins from the circulatory system into the tissues of the body. The increased thromboxane:prostacyclin ratio also results in the clumping together of platelets with corresponding coagulation abnormalities.

Signs and symptoms Because of the potential involvement of many of the organs of the body, the presenting signs and symptoms of pre-eclampsia can vary dramatically between individuals. It is essential therefore, that the midwife establishes a close relationship with the pregnant woman in order to recognize any changes in her condition. Often, the midwife who knows her woman well, will identify a potential problem without overt indications of a deterioration in her condition.

Classic signs of pre-eclampsia are a rising blood pressure, proteinuria, evidence of oedema, although this is not diagnostic, and subtle changes in blood chemistry. However, these signs are very individual and absence of hypertension does not rule out pre-eclampsia. Individual signs and symptoms depend on the organs and systems damaged by pre-eclampsia (see below).

Diagnosis There is no consistency in the diagnosis of pre-eclampsia. One widely accepted definition is an increase in diastolic blood pressure to >110 mmHg on one occasion or >90 mmHg on two or more occasions, 4 h apart, with proteinuria. However, an increase in diastolic blood pressure 15–20 mmHg above that at the booking visit with protein in the urine is also considered to indicate pre-eclampsia. Systolic blood pressure is an indication of cardiac output; diastolic blood pressure is however more affected by peripheral resistance. Thus, diastolic blood pressure is more diagnostic in pre-eclampsia.

NB: Because of cardiovascular changes related to pregnancy and pre-eclampsia, automated blood pressure monitors systematically underestimate blood pressure in pregnancy and should be used with caution (Duley et al 2006).

Oedema may be present but is not considered to be one of the cardinal signs of pre-eclampsia as it is found in the majority of pregnancies (Davies et al 2002). Proteinuria is measured accurately by

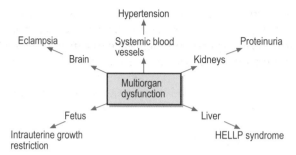

Figure 2.5 Principal organs affected by pre-eclampsia.

24 h urine collection. This result plus other laboratory tests for liver function, coagulation factors, full blood count and uric acid levels give a clear indication of the severity of the condition.

Pathological changes to body systems As indicated with the discussion on the pathophysiology of the condition, pre-eclampsia results in multisystem dysfunction (Fig. 2.5). Many vulnerable organs are likely to be damaged by generalized vasospasm and endothelial damage brought about by the release of toxins by the ischaemic placenta:

- Renal damage: The kidneys are particularly sensitive to hypertension. The increased pressure of the blood entering the Bowman's capsule results in damage to the endothelial cells of the glomerular filter. Proteins leak out in the filtrate resulting in proteinuria. Vasospasm of the afferent arterioles decreases blood flow into the kidneys preventing adequate excretion of waste products. Creatinine and uric acid are retained in the blood and levels rise indicating renal damage. Oliguria is a late and serious indication of organ damage and worsening pre-eclampsia.

- Liver damage: Vasoconstriction results in hypoxia of the cells of the liver. Liver cells become necrosed and this is indicated by the presence of liver enzymes such as aspartate transaminase in the blood. Damage to the endothelial cells of the blood vessels in the liver result in the leakage of fluid into the tissues of the liver. Resulting oedema in the liver ultimately causes pain as the liver swells within the liver capsule. This is experienced by the woman as epigastric pain and must be considered in any woman complaining of 'indigestion'.

- Cerebral damage: Similar changes occur in the brain, resulting in oedema and cerebral haemorrhage. Initially, the woman will complain of frontal headache. This may however lead to convulsions – eclampsia. In severe hypertension, cerebral vasospasm with oedema and thrombosis may result in encephalopathy.

- Pulmonary damage: Vascular damage may result in loss of proteins and fluid into the substance of the lungs. This may be compounded by fluid replacement therapy during treatment for pre-eclampsia and prevention of eclampsia. Additionally, cardiac compromise due to hypertension and the extra effort required by the heart to pump blood through the constricted systemic circulation may result in pulmonary congestion.

- Vision: Vasoconstriction in the retina may result in blurred vision or photophobia. Hypertension may also result in damage to the delicate blood vessels of the retina causing minute haemorrhages, which interfere with function. The woman may complain of visual disturbances.

- Haematological changes: With movement of fluid into interstitial tissues, circulating blood will become more concentrated increasing the haematocrit and haemoglobin levels. Damage to the endothelial lining of the blood vessels will result in the activation of the coagulation pathway resulting in abnormal coagulation studies. As this is widespread within the body, platelets are quickly used up. Thrombocytopenia results. Additionally, fibrin is being deposited within the blood vessels along with platelets – over time, this will occlude the vessels preventing blood reaching organs and systems of the body.

- Placental insufficiency: As a consequence of the maladaptation of the spiral arteries feeding the placenta, blood flow to the placenta is reduced. As the spiral arteries retain their muscular layer, these blood vessels are affected by the normal hormonal adjustments going on within the body as a whole. This will allow vasoconstriction and further reduction in blood flow. Uterine blood flow is also reduced due to hypertension. Placental tissue becomes ischaemic and infarctions occur. Placental function is compromised.

Management of hypertensive disorders of pregnancy Dealing with the hypertensive disorders of pregnancy as discrete disease processes is not straightforward, as management depends more on the effects of the pathophysiology than on its cause. Indeed, many pathologists suggest a common pathogenesis for these conditions (Ray et al 2005). Higgins & de Swiet (2001) suggest that basing a definition of pre-eclampsia on hypertension and proteinuria ignores the clinical variability of the condition. They suggest that the condition pre-eclampsia should be assumed in the absence of proteinuria but when hypertension and other severe symptoms, such as headache, thrombocytopenia or fetal compromise, are present. Management will therefore be discussed for pre-eclampsia but it should be understood that this applies to PIH and essential hypertension when pathology is similar.

The goal of management of a woman with pre-eclampsia is to prevent convulsions, control blood pressure and deliver the woman and her fetus safely. CEMACH (Lewis & Drife 2004) recommends that because of the difficulty with diagnosis and management of this condition, all obstetric units should have clear, written management protocols for severe pre-eclampsia to guide initial and ongoing treatment in hospital.

Management depends on the severity of the condition. Any woman who is found to have hypertension with proteinuria needs thorough assessment. Maternal and fetal condition must be assessed fully. Provided there is no indication of a worsening condition, regular monitoring as a day patient is indicated. Delivery of the placenta will ultimately resolve the condition.

Prevention Good prenatal care will identify those at greatest risk, including those less likely to attend for prenatal care (Duckitt & Harrington 2005). A planned programme of prenatal care can then be initiated with the multidisciplinary team. However, there is as yet no method of preventing these disorders and thus careful surveillance is the basis of management with early detection of the conditions.

The use of aspirin is still under debate. Aspirin is thought to prevent the production of thromboxane. The CLASP trial (1994) concluded that low dose aspirin might be beneficial for those women at high risk of early onset pre-eclampsia. Additionally, a later systematic review considers low dose aspirin commenced early in pregnancy to be associated with a 15% reduction in the risk of pre-eclampsia, a 14% reduction in the risks of a stillbirth or neonatal death and an 8% reduction in pre-term birth (Duley et al 2001).

Prenatal care There is debate at present regarding the frequency of prenatal visits, with some research suggesting that the accepted pattern of care, monthly until 28 weeks, bi-weekly to 36 weeks and weekly until birth, is unnecessary. An argument against this is that many cases of pre-eclampsia arise in women who have not been identified as at-risk of the condition and therefore less frequent prenatal visits would put these women at increased risk. However, pre-eclampsia often develops rapidly and within days of an antenatal assessment and thus it is essential that women are made aware of the symptoms of pre-eclampsia and the need for regular assessment (Greer 2005).

Any woman with one of the predisposing factors listed above should be offered specialist input before 20 weeks' gestation (Milne et al 2005). Prenatal care will include observation of the two principal features of the hypertensive disorders, blood pressure measurement and urinalysis. A baseline blood pressure will be carried out at the booking visit and any rise identified at each prenatal visit (Box 2.3). Presence of protein in the urine will require further investigation to identify if this is due to infection or contamination, or is a sign of hypertension or one of its complications. Weighing women prenatally is not normally carried out nowadays and observation of oedema is not an accurate indication of pre-eclampsia.

In any woman in whom there are indications of the development of hypertension or pre-eclampsia, laboratory tests can be carried out to identify pathological changes to the organs and systems of the body.

Treatment depends on the severity of the condition. However, it is extremely difficult to define severity based on blood pressure measurements or urinalysis. Laboratory tests are the best gauge of this and the health of the fetus is also crucial to the decisions made regarding treatment. Regular abdominal examination will identify growth and

Box 2.3 Blood pressure measurement

When using a conventional sphygmomanometer, there can be a variation in measurement as a result of either instrument error or observer error. Instrument error may be caused by an incorrectly calibrated or damaged manometer. All such equipment must be regularly serviced. Observer error can be considerable. Observation skills, such as reaction time and concentration, vary between individuals. Poor technique is, however, one factor that can be easily corrected.

Correct blood pressure measurement can be achieved by ensuring the following:

- The cuff should be placed at the level of the heart
- The cuff should be the correct size for the patient
- In pregnancy, the woman should be seated or propped up at a 45° angle (Fig. 2.6)
- Diastolic measurement should be taken at Korotkoff phase V (Table 2.1)
- Blood pressure measurement should be estimated to the nearest 2 mmHg.

Table 2.1 Korotkoff sounds

Phase	Audible sound
I	Clear tapping sound
II	Less clear murmur or swishing sound
III	Clear sound returns
IV	Muffling of sound
V	Disappearance of sound

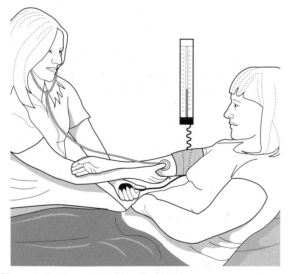

Figure 2.6 Correct position for blood pressure measurement.

fetal movement. A biophysical profile will be undertaken regularly. This includes the use of kick charts, cardiotocograph and ultrasound, looking at fetal growth, liquor volume and breathing movements with Doppler analysis of umbilical artery blood flow (Morley 2004). Based on all the above information, a decision will be made regarding treatment, which will be reviewed at frequent intervals.

Mild to moderate pre-eclampsia Mild or moderate pre-eclampsia can usually be controlled by rest and a stress free lifestyle. Resting in a lateral recumbent position takes the pressure of the gravid uterus off the inferior vena cava and increases circulatory volume. Blood pressure normally drops as a result, enhancing blood flow to the placenta and fetus (Gilbert & Harmon 1998). However, the risks associated with bed rest must be weighed against any benefit (see Ch. 4). The use of antihypertensives in women with a diastolic pressure <100 mmHg has been shown to be of little benefit to either mother or the fetus in this group of women (Abalos et al 2007). A good diet is recommended; rich in calcium and omega three supplementation, both of which are beneficial to pregnant women.

During this time, the medical team must plan care in partnership with the woman who probably feels well and wonders what the fuss is all about. The midwife's social and psychological skills will be vital in managing this woman and her family. Good communication skills by all concerned are essential.

Rest at home and regular visits by the midwife may be all that is required in these cases. Bed rest will improve blood flow to all organs of the body and minimize ischaemia. Day care in an assessment unit may be recommended periodically to undertake a more thorough examination of both the woman and her baby by undertaking cardiotocography, blood tests, ultrasound and Doppler studies. Careful monitoring of proteinuria may give some indication of the severity of the condition.

Severe pre-eclampsia Severe pre-eclampsia occurs in 0.5% of all pregnant women (RCOG 2006) and is indicated by a blood pressure >160/110 mmHg and the presence of significant proteinuria. Laboratory tests will indicate involvement of the liver and increasing damage to the kidneys by the presence of liver enzymes and >0.3 g of protein in a 24 h collection of urine. A rise in uric acid levels in particular relates to a poor outcome for mother and baby (Martin et al 1999). At this stage, the multidisciplinary team is faced with the dilemma of expediting delivery at a time when the fetus is as mature as possible but without risking serious damage to the woman.

Clinical warning signs of severe pre-eclampsia in addition to hypertension and proteinuria are (RCOG 2006):

- Severe headache
- Visual disturbances
- Epigastric pain or vomiting
- Signs of clonus
- Papilloedema
- Liver tenderness
- Platelet count <100 × 10⁶/L
- Abnormal liver enzymes (ALT or AST >70 IU/L)
- HELLP syndrome.

The use of antihypertensives is a difficult decision for the team. One reason for the increase in blood pressure is to ensure an adequate circulation to the placenta and fetus. Artificial lowering of the blood pressure may seriously prevent the fetus receiving sufficient nutrients and oxygen. Ultrasound measurement of fetal growth will be essential to identify any compromise. However, the deaths of nine women in the recent CEMACH report from a cerebral vascular accident (Lewis & Drife 2004) indicate a failure of effective antihypertensive therapy and thus this must be initiated where appropriate.

Labetalol is commonly the antihypertensive of choice, as this can be given orally initially and subsequently intravenously if required. However, labetalol should not be used in a woman with asthma. Other useful antihypertensive drugs include oral nifedipine or intravenous hydralazine (RCOG 2006). The use of antihypertensive drugs may assist in prolonging the pregnancy to

> **Box 2.4 Lung maturation**
>
> Before birth, fetal lungs are filled with fluid and respiratory function is carried out by the placenta. At birth, the lungs expand and fill with air. One vital component of this process is the presence of surfactant. Surfactant is a phospholipid which lowers surface tension of the walls of the alveoli preventing their collapse with each expiration. Surfactant is produced from 23 weeks' gestation but there is insufficient present to prevent alveolar collapse until 28–30 weeks' gestation.
>
> A fetus who is born during these early weeks will develop respiratory distress syndrome (RDS). In those whose birth is anticipated, the administration of a glucocorticoid, such as betamethasone for 24–48 h, will speed up the production of surfactant and thus substantially reduce the incidence of RDS.

the benefit of the fetus. If the fetus is <34 weeks' gestation, corticosteroids can be administered to reduce fetal respiratory complications (Box 2.4).

Anticonvulsant prophylaxis may be considered. Magnesium sulphate has been shown to be more effective than either phenytoin or diazepam in severe pre-eclampsia (Eclampsia Trial Collaborative Group 1995). In the Magpie Trial, magnesium sulphate was found to halve the risk of eclampsia and was found to be beneficial in preventing maternal death (Magpie Trial Collaborative Group 2002). Magnesium is required for metabolism, smooth muscle control and nerve function. Increased levels of magnesium in the body depress the activity of all excitable tissue. It is thought that magnesium prevents/treats eclampsia by relieving spasm of cerebral blood vessels, thus improving perfusion of tissue. It is also thought to protect the endothelium of blood vessels from damage by free radicals.

Administration of magnesium sulphate must be carefully monitored, as raised levels are highly toxic to the body. This is aggravated if renal function is impaired as magnesium is eliminated by the kidneys. Magnesium toxicity leads to respiratory depression and loss of deep tendon reflexes. Calcium gluconate will reverse this toxicity.

Treatment in labour Labour increases the risks to both mother and fetus. Both must be closely monitored and the mother observed for rising blood pressure, falling urinary output and increasing proteinuria. Careful observation of fluid balance is essential as the woman with pre-eclampsia is volume depleted, with low cardiac output, low pulmonary pressure and high systemic peripheral resistance. Cardiac function may be compromised giving rise to pulmonary oedema, adult respiratory distress syndrome (ARDS) or a cerebrovascular accident (stroke). Pulse oximetry can be useful as it gives an early indication of pulmonary oedema. It may be necessary to insert a central line and measure central venous pressure with expert advice on the use of fluids. Use of Syntocinon must be monitored carefully because Syntocinon is a diuretic causing further imbalance. Plasma expanders may be required to attract fluid back into the circulatory system and reduce oedema in vital organs such as the brain, lungs and liver.

Pain management is essential to reduce psychological stress. An epidural is ideal as long as coagulation studies are satisfactory. The advantages of an epidural are that it can increase placental blood flow by up to 75%, it decreases and stabilizes maternal blood pressure, does not cause respiratory depression, and provides excellent analgesia. Again, careful fluid balance is essential.

Continuous fetal monitoring is also mandatory. The fetus may already be compromised by the effects of hypertension and other consequences of pre-eclampsia, such as intrauterine growth restriction, placental insufficiency and prematurity.

The second stage of labour may be shortened by instrumental delivery depending on progress. Directed pushing is not advised, as this can produce increased pressures which may exacerbate the effects of pre-eclampsia.

In the third stage, ergometrine is contraindicated, as this causes peripheral vasoconstriction which would increase hypertension. Intravenous Syntocinon is the drug of choice.

Postnatal All observations must continue after delivery until it can be seen that the condition is improving. Cardiac load will increase in the first 24–48 h after delivery, due to the return of uterine blood to the systemic circulation. Thus, blood pressure will fall immediately postpartum but will rise after 24 h, peaking 2–4 days postpartum (Jordan 2002). Some 44% of eclamptic fits occur postpartum and thus close observation must continue (Lubarsky et al 1994). Antihypertensive therapy is considered safe during breast-feeding.

COMPLICATIONS OF HYPERTENSIVE DISORDERS OF PREGNANCY

Fulminating pre–eclampsia

This condition, although rare, can be life-threatening to both mother and baby. Typically, the woman is well until, without warning, she develops severe pre-eclampsia over a few hours or days. Prenatal women and their families should be educated about pre-eclampsia, as they may not realize the seriousness of this rapidly developing condition.

Eclampsia

Eclampsia is a condition in which a woman, who may or may not have been diagnosed with one of the hypertensive disorders, suffers a fit similar to that of a grand mal epileptic seizure. This is a major crisis for the woman and also for her fetus if the seizure occurs prenatally or during labour. Ventilation ceases during the seizure and thus the already compromised fetus is at considerable risk of hypoxia.

Eclampsia occurs in 1 in 2000–3000 births in developed countries (Mattar & Sibai 2000) and carries a high maternal and fetal mortality. Eclampsia may occur prenatally, intranatally, or postnatally. The postnatal period is the time of greatest risk (Lubarsky et al 1994). Eclampsia occurs as a consequence of cerebral hypoxia from oedema and the presence of small haemorrhages caused by hypertension or vascular damage. This causes dysfunction of the neural pathways resulting in convulsions.

As in epilepsy, the seizure has four stages:

1. Premonitory stage: Often missed unless closely watched. Twitching of facial muscles or rolling of eyes may be seen.

2. Tonic stage: Violent prolonged spasm of muscles, including respiratory muscles thus resulting in cyanosis.
3. Clonic stage: Muscular jerking movements of relatively short duration.
4. Coma: Unconsciousness will ensue often with noisy breathing. This stage can last for several hours.

Prognosis

Eclampsia is a major obstetric emergency. Death occurs from cerebral haemorrhage, pulmonary oedema, ARDS, renal or liver failure. If not controlled, repeated fits (*status eclampticus*) may result in cardiac failure. The fetus, already compromised by placental insufficiency, and possibly hypoxia, will be seriously affected by each successive fit and may die in utero.

Treatment

Any woman with severe pre-eclampsia is at risk of having an eclamptic fit. Both prevention and treatment is by intravenous infusion with magnesium sulphate, as discussed above. The initial dose is as a bolus intravenous injection of 4–5 g in saline or dextrose slowly over 15–20 min, then as a continuous infusion of 1–2 g/h (Jordan 2002). Careful monitoring must be carried out as magnesium sulphate toxicity may occur. This can be seen as muscle paralysis, respiratory and cardiac arrest. The antidote calcium gluconate must be available at all times. This is administered as 10 ml of 10% calcium gluconate over 3–5 min.

This woman must be carefully monitored for complications, such as renal failure, liver failure, disseminated intravascular coagulation (DIC) or HELLP syndrome.

HELLP syndrome (Haemolysis, Elevated Liver enzymes, Low Platelets)

The hypertensive disorders of pregnancy cover a spectrum of disease processes. HELLP syndrome is a variant of pre-eclampsia and is associated with considerable cardiopulmonary morbidity and mortality (Terrone et al 2000). This condition, although rare, carries a high mortality and

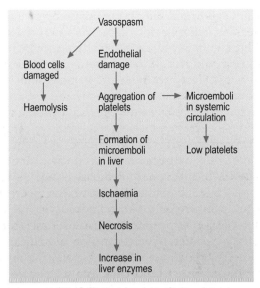

Figure 2.7   Pathological process of HELLP syndrome.

morbidity rate. Mortality rate has been variously reported as between 2–24%.

HELLP syndrome typically manifests itself between 32 and 34 weeks' gestation but it should be noted that 30% of cases occur postpartum (Lloyd 2003). HELLP syndrome shows a similar pathology to DIC but usually has normal prothrombin times. Changes that are evident however, are (Fig. 2.7):

- Haemolysis: Vasospasm causes damage to the endothelium of blood vessels which will then damage blood cells as they pass through the roughened vessels. Damaged blood cells are normally destroyed by the body and replaced – haemolysis. Large-scale destruction of blood cells will however prevent normal physiological processes occurring, such as transportation of oxygen. Hyperbilirubinaemia (jaundice) may develop as a result of increased haemolysis
- Liver damage, as described above, will result in the release of liver enzymes into the bloodstream thus elevating serum liver enzymes
- Platelets are used up as a result of inappropriate production of microemboli throughout the body, thus resulting in low serum platelet levels.

HELLP syndrome may occur suddenly or insidiously. The majority of women with this condition present with severe epigastric pain; 50% have vomiting and 80% have hypertension (Terrone et al 2000). However, it should be noted that 20% of women with this condition are normotensive. Oedema may be present. Other symptoms may include haematuria, gastrointestinal bleeding, viral symptoms and proteinuria.

Differential diagnosis is thus confusing. The disorder may be diagnosed as conditions such as gastroenteritis, pancreatitis or cholecystitis. However, any pregnant woman with epigastric pain, nausea and vomiting, or pre-eclampsia, must have serum liver enzymes and platelets measured to rule out a hypertensive complication.

Management of the condition is very difficult. The woman should be transferred to a high dependency unit for intravenous fluid hydration with albumin, fresh frozen plasma and platelets. Anticonvulsants, antihypertensives and diuretics may be required. Delivery will be expedited. This will be an extremely worrying time for the woman and her family and time should be taken to explain the situation carefully.

Midwifery management

Midwives are the lead practitioners in the majority of pregnancies and must be alert for risk factors and the development of hypertension in pregnancy. Planned antenatal care, including an increased number of antenatal visits in those at risk, will increase the likelihood of detecting hypertension quickly. The midwife should also be alert for signs of pre-eclampsia even in those women who are normotensive, and be aware that proteinuria is serious with or without hypertension. *It is essential that urine is tested for protein for all women at every prenatal visit* (Lewis & Drife 2004).

One vital role for the midwife is to ensure that pregnant women and their families are educated about these conditions. Action on Pre-eclampsia (APEC) is a support group whose aim it is to educate the public and health professionals about this and associated conditions as they recognize that few women realize how dangerous the condition is to themselves and their babies.

Women will be assessed in a day care provision where possible; however, women suffering from severe pre-eclampsia will be admitted to hospital where they will be closely monitored in a high dependency unit, while a decision is made about delivery.

If the woman's condition warrants it, magnesium sulphate will be prescribed. The midwife must observe carefully for magnesium sulphate toxicity – early signs are thirst, warmth and flushing. Patellar reflexes will be tested regularly, particularly before each dose, as absence of reflexes indicates magnesium toxicity. Delivery will be induced once the woman's condition is stabilized. The paediatrician should be present at delivery because magnesium sulphate toxicity can occur in the neonate immediately post-delivery. Magnesium sulphate is usually discontinued gradually after 24–48h, having started the woman on another anticonvulsant, such as phenobarbital.

The midwife's role during this stressful time will be to carry out all observations and carefully document care. Essential treatments only will be carried out with minimal disturbance to minimize the risk of eclampsia. A vital component of the midwife's care will be to communicate effectively with the woman and her family, reassuring them and educating them in the plan of care.

Should the woman experience an eclamptic fit, the midwife will need to deal with this, as with any form of seizure. Principles of care will be to:

- Summon medical aid
- Maintain a clear airway by rolling her gently on to her side or placing a wedge under her left side if at all possible without injury to either the woman or the midwife
- Give oxygen as soon as possible
- Prevent injury by moving away any furniture or hazards, pulling up padded cot sides
- Document the time and length of the seizure.

Training of all healthcare workers in the management of an eclamptic fit, as with all obstetric emergencies, in the form of practice drills and on-site simulation has been shown to improve maternal and fetal outcome (Thompson et al 2004).

It is recommended that drug therapy should not be commenced until the initial fit is over, unless the patient has an intravenous infusion in situ. Care must be taken not to prescribe poly-pharmacy in an attempt to arrest the fit, as this can lead to respiratory arrest. Immediately after the fit, appropriate medication can be initiated to prevent status eclampticus.

During the seizure, the woman will become hypoxic as respiratory muscles will be affected by the muscle spasm. Fetal well-being must be monitored immediately the seizure has ceased. A cardiotocograph should be commenced and remain in situ until delivery is expedited.

The woman will be moved to a high dependency area for close monitoring and she will remain comatose for some time after the seizure. The midwife's role will be to record vital signs at frequent intervals and document all care. Fluid intake and output will be carefully monitored. The midwife should be alert for signs that labour has commenced, by regular abdominal examination.

Other aspects of a midwife's care are to observe for further deterioration, such as the onset of DIC or HELLP syndrome by observing for inappropriate bleeding from wounds, nose or mouth. Renal function will be assessed by hourly urine output via an indwelling catheter.

Prognosis

It may take up to 3 months for a woman to become normotensive after suffering from pre-eclampsia in pregnancy. In addition, it has been shown that these women are at increased risk of developing cardiovascular complications later in life (Ramsay et al 2003). Women with pre-existing hypertension and those who develop pregnancy-induced hypertension will be advised to have their condition monitored closely to prevent complications, such as renal disease, developing.

Future pregnancies

One study looking at each of the hypertensive disorders in a first pregnancy found a 20–50%

occurrence rate in a second pregnancy; 19% of those with PIH, 32% with pre-eclampsia and 46% with essential hypertension (Zhang et al 2001). The earlier the onset of hypertension in the first pregnancy, the higher the overall recurrence rate. Women who have had hypertensive disorders in pregnancy therefore should be advised of these risks before considering a subsequent pregnancy. They should also be assessed for underlying pathology. Evidence suggests that up to 13% of women with pre-eclampsia will have an underlying essential hypertension that was not suspected prenatally (Wilson et al 2003).

The neonate

Hypertensive disorders of pregnancy are leading causes of fetal and neonatal morbidity and mortality worldwide. Women with hypertensive disease in pregnancy are at significantly higher risk of having pregnancies complicated by infants who are small for gestational age or stillborn, in comparison with women with normotensive pregnancies (Allen et al 2004).

The baby whose mother required magnesium sulphate should be observed closely for the first 48h, as this substance causes respiratory depression in the neonate. High levels of magnesium can result in apnoea, especially if magnesium was administered within 2h of birth. Respiratory depression caused by magnesium is not easily reversed and the neonate will require intensive care facilities. Drug interactions are potentially dangerous and these must also be considered in the care of both mother and infant.

High levels of magnesium cause drowsiness and breast-feeding may need to be delayed by 24h to allow the majority of the excess magnesium to be eliminated from the neonate. With extra support, the mother, if well enough, should be encouraged to care for her infant and express her milk during this time.

Support group

Action on Pre-eclampsia (APEC) – www.apec.org.uk

REFERENCES

Abalos E, Duley L, Steyn D W, Henderson-Smart D J 2007 Antihypertensive drug therapy for mild to moderate hypertension in pregnancy. Cochrane Database of Systematic Reviews. Issue 1. Art No: CD002252

Allen V M, Joseph K S, Murphy K E, Magee L A, Ohlsson A 2004 The effect of hypertensive disorders in pregnancy on small for gestational age and stillbirth: a population based study. BMC Pregnancy and Childbirth 4:17–25

Atallah A, Hofmeyr G, Duley L 2006 Calcium supplementation during pregnancy for preventing hypertensive disorders and related problems Cochrane Database of Systematic Reviews. Issue 3. Art No: CD001059

Beevers G, Lip G Y H, O'Brien E 2001 ABC of hypertension: The pathophysiology of hypertension. British Medical Journal 322:912–916

Blackburn S 2002 Maternal, fetal and neonatal physiology: A clinical perspective, 2nd edn. WB Saunders, Philadelphia, p 255–309

CLASP Collaborative Group 1994 CLASP; a randomized trial of low dose aspirin for the prevention and treatment of pre-eclampsia among 9364 pregnant women. Lancet 343(8898):619–632

Davies L, Waugh J, Kilby M 2002 Assessing proteinuria in hypertensive pregnancy. British Journal of Midwifery 10(7): 441–445

Duckett R A, Kenny L, Baker P N 2001 Hypertension in pregnancy. Current Obstetrics and Gynaecology 11(1):7–14

Duckitt K, Harrington D 2005 Risk factors for pre-eclampsia at antenatal booking: systematic review of controlled studies. British Medical Journal 330(7491):565–571

Duley L, Henderson-Smart D, Knight M, King J 2001 Antiplatelet drugs for prevention of pre-eclampsia and its consequences: systematic review. British Medical Journal 322(7282):329–333

Duley L, Meher S, Abalos E 2006 Management of pre-eclampsia. British Medical Journal 332(7539):463–468

Eclampsia Trial Collaborative Group 1995 Which anticonvulsant with eclampsia? Evidence for the Collaborative Eclampsia Trial. Lancet 345:1455–1463

Gilbert E S, Harmon J S 1998 High risk pregnancy and delivery. Mosby, St Louis, p 489–539

Greer I A 2005 Pre-eclampsia matters. British Medical Journal 330:549–550

Gutierrez K J, Petersen P G 2002 Pathophysiology. WB Saunders, Philadelphia, p 111

Higgins J R, de Swiet M 2001 Blood pressure measurement and classification in pregnancy. Lancet 357(9250):131–135

Jordan S 2002 Pharmacology for midwives. Palgrave, Houndmills, p 223–253

Kennedy S 2002 Review of current management of essential hypertension. Nursing and Residential Care 4(12):582–585

Koelman C, Coumans A, Nijman H et al 2000 Correlation between oral sex and a low incidence of pre-eclampsia: a role for soluble HLA in seminal fluid. Journal of Reproductive Immunology 46(2):155–166

Lewis G, Drife J (eds) 2004 Why Mothers Die 2000–2002: The sixth report of the Confidential Enquires into Maternal Deaths in the United Kingdom. RCOG, London

Lloyd C 2003 Common medical disorders associated with pregnancy. In: Fraser DM, Cooper MA (eds) Myles textbook for midwives. Churchill Livingstone, Edinburgh, p 321–355

Lubarsky S L, Barton J R, Friedman S A et al 1994 Late postpartum eclampsia revisited. Obstetrics and Gynaecology 83:502–505

Magee L A 2001 Treating hypertension in women of childbearing age and during pregnancy. Drug Safety 14(6):457–474

Magpie Trial Collaborative Group 2002 Do women with pre-eclampsia, and their babies, benefit from magnesium sulphate? The Magpie trial: a randomized placebo-controlled trial. Lancet 359:1877–1890

Martin J N Jr, May W L, Magann E F et al 1999 Early risk assessment of severe pre-eclampsia: admission battery of symptoms and laboratory tests to predict likelihood of subsequent significant maternal morbidity. American Journal of Obstetrics and Gynecology 180:1407–1414

Mattar F, Sibai B M 2000 Eclampsia VIII: Risk factors for maternal morbidity. American Journal of Obstetrics and Gynecology 182(2):307–312

Milne F, Redman C, Walker J et al 2005 The pre-eclampsia community guideline (PRECOG): how to screen for and detect onset of pre-eclampsia in the community. British Medical Journal 330(7491):576–580

Morley A 2004 Pre-eclampsia: pathophysiology and its management British Journal of Midwifery 12(1):30–37

Murray I 2003 Change and adaptation in pregnancy. In: Frazer DM, Cooper MA (eds) Myles' Textbook for Midwives, 14th edn. Churchill Livingstone, Edinburgh, p 185–213

Ramsay J E, Stewart F, Green I A, Sattar N 2003 Microvascular dysfunction: a link between pre-eclampsia and maternal coronary heart disease. British Journal of Obstetrics and Gynaecology 110:1029–1031

Ray J G, Vermeulen M J, Schull M J, Redelmeier D A 2005 Cardiovascular health after maternal placental syndromes (CHAMPS): population-based retrospective cohort study. Lancet 366(9499):1797–1803

RCOG 2006 The management of severe pre-eclampsia/eclampsia. Guideline No 10(A). RCOG, London

Redman C W G, Sargent I L 2001 The pathogenesis of pre-eclampsia. Gynecologie Obstetrique & Fertilite 29(7–8):518–522

Robinson J 2004 Toenails and selenium: preventing pre-eclampsia. British Journal of Midwifery 12(6):366

Soydemir F, Kenny L 2006 Hypertension in pregnancy. Current Opinion in Obstetrics and Gynecology 16:315–320

Terrone D A, Isler C M, May W L, Magann E F, Norman P F, Martin J N Jr 2000 Cardiopulmonary morbidity as a complication of severe preeclampsia HELLP syndrome Journal of Perinatology 2:78–81

Thompson S, Neal S, Clark V 2004 Clinical risk management in obstetric eclamptic drills. British Medical Journal 328(7434):269–271

Wilson B J, Watson M S, Prescott G J et al 2003 Hypertensive diseases of pregnancy and risk of hypertension and strokes in later life: results from a cohort study. British Medical Journal 326(7394):845–851

Zhang J, Troendle J F, Levine R J 2001 Risks of hypertensive disorders in the second pregnancy. Paediatric and Perinatal Epidemiology 15(3):226–231

Chapter 3

Cardiac conditions

INTRODUCTION

It is rare in industrialized countries to see young people debilitated by a cardiac problem. Those who have a congenital defect at birth will in most cases have had surgery to correct the problem. Rheumatic fever which damages the heart in children and adults is virtually unheard of. However, there remains a small proportion of women of childbearing age who have a known defect that has caused no problems to date and has not required treatment. There are also some women in whom a defect has been corrected and some in whom one has not been diagnosed. For these women, pregnancy and childbirth can be dangerous depending on how well the damaged heart can deal with the extra workload.

Although cardiac disease in pregnancy complicates few pregnancies, it continues to contribute significantly to maternal and fetal mortality and morbidity. Some 10–25% of all maternal deaths are due to cardiac disease (Avila et al 2003). The main causes of maternal mortality are: pulmonary hypertension, endocarditis, cardiomyopathy, myocarditis, coronary artery disease and sudden lethal cardiac arrhythmia. Medical advances have increased the number of women who survive to adulthood and successfully achieve pregnancy. The midwife must therefore have a good understanding of these disorders in order to care for them appropriately.

RELEVANT ANATOMY AND PHYSIOLOGY

The heart is a cone-shaped muscular hollow organ situated in a space between the lungs – the mediastinum (Fig. 3.1). The muscular wall is composed of an outer protective layer, the pericardium, a middle muscular layer, the myocardium and an innermost layer – the endocardium. The *pericardium* is a double outermost layer which surrounds the heart preventing overfilling and also allowing free movement within the mediastinum. The muscular *myocardium* varies in thickness reflecting the work required by the underlying chamber of the heart. The endothelial *endocardium* lines the heart, the valves and the blood vessels leaving the heart and provides a smooth surface reducing friction between blood and the walls of the heart.

The four chambers of the heart: the right and left atria (singular atrium) and right and left ventricles, are separated by valves which prevent the blood flowing backwards into the heart. With each contraction of the heart, all four valves open and allow blood to pass through. As the heart relaxes, these valves close and it is the sounds of the valves closing that create the familiar 'lub-dup' heart sounds heard through a stethoscope.

The four valves of the heart are:

1. The tricuspid valve, situated between the right atrium and ventricle, composed of three flaps or cusps
2. The mitral valve, between the left atrium and ventricle. This valve is also known as the bicuspid valve as it is composed of two cusps
3. & 4. Two semilunar valves which are situated in the pulmonary artery and aorta as they leave the heart. These valves consist of three semicircular cusps attached to the inner surface of the heart.

The mitral and tricuspid valves are prevented from opening backwards into the atria by fibres – the chordae tendineae, attached to the walls of the ventricles.

Deoxygenated blood from the body enters the right atrium of the heart via the vena cava (Fig. 3.2). Once the atrium is filled, the tricuspid valve opens and, assisted by contraction of the atria, the blood is moved into the right ventricle. Once this has filled, the ventricle contracts and pushes the blood into the pulmonary arteries. Blood is carried to the lungs where it is oxygenated and then returned to the left side of the heart. In synchrony with the right side, oxygenated blood pours into

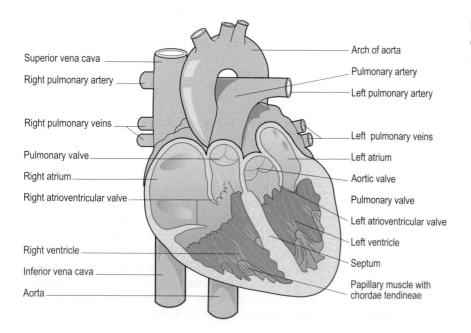

Figure 3.1   Internal structure of the heart.

Superior vena cava

Right pulmonary artery

Right pulmonary veins

Pulmonary valve

Right atrium

Right atrioventricular valve

Right ventricle

Inferior vena cava

Aorta

Arch of aorta

Pulmonary artery

Left pulmonary artery

Left pulmonary veins

Left atrium

Aortic valve

Pulmonary valve

Left atrioventricular valve

Left ventricle

Septum

Papillary muscle with chordae tendineae

the left atrium, is moved into the left ventricle and then into the aorta, the largest artery in the body. The heart then rests for a brief moment of time. The entire cycle – the cardiac cycle – takes 0.8 s and is controlled by the pacemaker of the heart.

PHYSIOLOGICAL CHANGES IN PREGNANCY

Prenatally cardiac output increases from the first trimester until it reaches a plateau at 28–34 weeks. This is due to the increase in blood volume, the effects of the hormones of pregnancy and the increase in vasculature through the uterus. These alterations increase the workload of the heart considerably but healthy women are able to adjust to these physiological changes with ease (see also Ch. 2). However, the changes provoke symptoms similar to mild cardiac disease such as dyspnoea, especially with exercise, fatigue and oedema. Additionally, the above changes may provoke the occasional dysrhythmia or episode of palpitations (Jordan 2002). There is also an increased risk of thromboembolism during pregnancy with the risk being highest after birth (Lee 2005).

During labour there is a significant increase in cardiac output as a result of uterine contractions and following birth blood returning from the uterine circulation increases blood volume dramatically until a brisk diuresis corrects fluid balance.

CARDIAC DISEASE IN PREGNANCY

The presence of heart disease although rare, is associated with a significant risk to mother and fetus. In the most recent Confidential Enquiry into Maternal and Child Health (CEMACH) 2000–2002, cardiac disease was the leading cause of indirect death with 44 mortalities in the 3 years (Lewis & Drife 2004). Cardiac disease was the second most common cause of maternal death overall, second only to psychiatric causes and more frequent than thromboembolic disease. In women with congenital heart disease, the presence of pulmonary hypertension was the crucial factor. In acquired disorders, the main causes were cardiomyopathy, myocardial infarction, aneurysm and dissection of the aorta. Eisenmenger's syndrome, although rare, is a life-threatening condition in pregnancy, carrying a 40% mortality rate with each pregnancy

Cardiac disorders are classified as congenital or acquired. In women of childbearing age, acquired disorders are rare. The most common cause of an acquired cardiac disorder in fertile women is rheumatic heart disease as a complication of rheumatic fever as a child. Congenital heart disease is more common in the UK (Iserin 2001) and occurs in 0.5–2% of the population (Gilbert & Harmon 1998).

Pathophysiology of cardiac disease

Acquired cardiac disorders

Acquired cardiac disorders occur as a complication of another disease process. In women of childbearing age, the cause of the damage may be scarring left after an inflammatory response to an infection. Although this is uncommon in the UK today, the most likely disease process is rheumatic fever. Other inflammatory conditions that rarely occur are infective endocarditis and pericarditis. Ischaemic heart disease in pregnancy is increasing, especially in women over the age of 34 years.

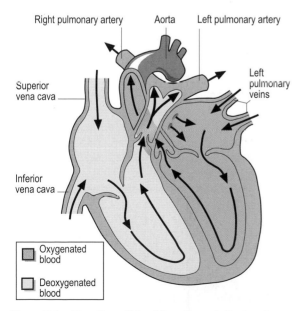

Figure 3.2 Direction of blood flow through the heart.

Rheumatic heart disease

Rheumatic heart disease is the result of an acute inflammatory complication of a group A streptococcus infection. This initial infection may present as a respiratory infection or scarlet fever. In people thought to be susceptible to the antibodies produced in the initial infection, rheumatic fever commonly manifests as fever and joint pain. The intensity of the fever can vary considerably however, from a mild condition that goes unnoticed to an acute illness with a mortality rate of 2–3%. A common complication of rheumatic fever is cardiac disease which may not show any symptoms for many years. Other organs that may be affected are the joints, skin and brain.

In those individuals with rheumatic heart disease, the endocardium becomes inflamed and subsequently scarred. This is found most commonly on the valves of the heart, particularly the mitral valve and to a lesser extent, the tricuspid valve. The valves become distorted and dysfunctional. The ends of the cusps of the valves become roughened, fuse together and the opening narrowed, a condition known as mitral or atrial (relating to the tricuspid valve) stenosis. Further, the damage may prevent the cusps of the valves from closing fully allowing backflow of blood in the heart, mitral/atrial incompetence. The result of these changes is a damaged heart in which circulation of blood is impaired (Box 3.1). The heart has to work harder to pump sufficient blood around the body. Over time, the heart increases in size, a condition known as hypertrophy. This weakens the heart and any further strain, such as pregnancy, may lead to heart failure.

Other conditions that have a similar effect are:

- Infective endocarditis: This is an inflammation of the endocardium of the heart particularly of the valves but from other infective disorders. Factors that predispose an individual to developing this condition include intravenous drug abuse, damaged valves (as described above), minor infections, dental treatment and cardiac surgery. In this condition, the infective organism grows on the valves scarring the tissue with similar results to rheumatic heart disease

- Pericarditis: This is inflammation of the pericardium as a result of infection, cardiac injury or an autoimmune response. This may result in pericardial infusion preventing the heart from expanding sufficiently, or scarring of the pericardium preventing stretch. The patient finds it painful to breathe and experiences chest pain.

Ischaemic heart disease and myocardial infarction

With increasing dietary and obesity problems in the industrialized world, it is becoming increasingly common to meet women who have the early signs of ischaemic heart disease. Blood vessels are damaged by a high level of circulating fats and plaques of atherosclerosis (Box 3.2) begin to narrow the lumen of the blood vessels (Foxton 2003). Where this happens in the coronary arteries surrounding and nourishing the tissues of the heart, the heart becomes ischaemic and is unable to continue functioning properly. Women are increasingly leaving pregnancy until they are older with the added risk that ischaemic heart disease may be well advanced. The added workload to the heart, of pregnancy and childbirth, may result in angina or rarely a heart attack – myocardial infarction (MI). Acute myocardial infarction during childbirth is very rare, occurring in 1 in 10 000–30 000 women (Baird & Kennedy 2006). However, maternal mortality from an MI may be up to 40%. Permanent changes to the heart due to chronic hypertension may also complicate pregnancy.

Box 3.1 Artificial valves

Surgery can significantly enlarge the size of an orifice bordered by an damaged heart valve. Some individuals however have too great a damage to the valve and require its replacement with an artificial valve. Artificial valves can be mechanical or tissue. Mechanical valves normally last for as long as required but the patient must take thromboprophylaxis for the rest of her life to prevent clots forming on the valve. A tissue valve does not require anticoagulants but does not last as long. Tissue valves, made traditionally from pig heart valves, are considered to last approximately 15 years.

Peripartum cardiomyopathy

This is a rare condition but one which carries a high mortality rate in pregnancy (Palmer 2006). Mortality rates range from 25–50%, with a significant number of deaths occurring shortly after the onset of symptoms (Lloyd 2003). It is a condition in which women with no previous history of heart disease develop enlargement and inflammation of the myocardium of the heart. The incidence is higher in older women and in those with hypertension.

Congenital heart disease

Congenital defects are the more common cause of heart disease in pregnancy. A structural defect present at birth will usually be identified in the UK and successful surgical treatment is increasing (Swinburne 2004). However, if this is not detected and the body is able to continue functioning normally, the individual may not show symptoms until added stress is put on the heart, as in pregnancy. Additionally, surgically corrected defects may not enable the heart to function at normal capacity and with the added workload of pregnancy, may also show symptoms for the first time.

The more common congenital defects seen in pregnancy include (Fig. 3.3):

- Atrial or ventricular septal defects
- Patent ductus arteriosus
- Pulmonary or aortic stenosis
- Syndromes such as Eisenmenger's and Marfan's.

Atrial or ventricular septal defects (ASD/VSD) are an abnormal opening between either the right and left atria or the right and left ventricle. In an unaffected heart, the left ventricle contains blood at higher pressure than the right because the left ventricle has to produce enough pressure to pump blood throughout the entire body. In the case of an ASD/VSD, blood therefore moves through the defect from the left to the right side of the heart. A small uncomplicated septal defect rarely causes any problems for women during pregnancy. However, over time and depending on many other factors, extra blood from the left atrium may cause a volume overload of both the right atrium and ventricle, which if left untreated, can result in enlargement of the right side of the heart and ultimately heart failure. Hypertension and coronary artery disease can aggravate this situation.

This constant overload of the right side of the heart will cause an overload of the entire pulmonary vasculature. Eventually the pulmonary vasculature will develop pulmonary hypertension to try to divert the extra blood volume away from the lungs. Over time, this causes changes in the lungs which will increase pressure in the right side of the heart. This will reverse the pressure gradient across the ASD, and the shunt will reverse; a right-to-left shunt will exist. This is known as *Eisenmenger's syndrome* a condition that carries a high mortality rate in pregnancy and childbirth. Women with this condition are therefore advised against pregnancy.

A *patent ductus arteriosus* is a remnant of fetal life. During pregnancy, blood is oxygenated by the placenta and the lungs are therefore not functioning. The fetal circulation is adapted to bypass the lungs by the presence of a temporary structure, the ductus arteriosus, between the pulmonary

---

Box 3.2 Atherosclerosis

Atherosclerosis is a disease affecting the arteries of the body. Commonly it is referred to as 'hardening' or 'furring' of the arteries, caused by the formation of multiple fatty plaques. Hardening refers to the changes in the blood vessel wall as a result of the presence of the plaques. Furring refers to the narrowing of the blood vessel preventing adequate blood supply to the organ it feeds.

Over a long period of time, the artery becomes more damaged until the vessel becomes completely occluded either by the plaques or by rupture of the plaque and the formation of a thrombus. This will often cause pain or dysfunction of the associated organ, such as a myocardial infarction if a coronary artery is involved, a cerebrovascular accident, 'stroke' if a cerebral artery is involved or other problems such as intermittent claudication, if one of the arteries of the legs is involved. Atherosclerosis is a bodywide process and can cause similar events anywhere in the body.

artery and the aorta. Rarely this structure does not close after birth. A patent ductus arteriosus allows oxygenated blood to flow down a pressure gradient from the aorta to the pulmonary arteries. Thus, some of the oxygenated blood does not reach the body, and the patient becomes short of breath and cyanotic. Pulmonary hypertension will also develop over time. Heart rate increases in an attempt to move sufficient blood to all areas of the body but if left untreated, the patient may develop heart failure. As with a septal defect, the degree of strain on the heart depends on how well the body copes with the added workload.

Pulmonary or aortic stenosis is a narrowing of the pulmonary artery or the aorta as it leaves the heart (Box 3.3). Movement of blood into the pulmonary or systemic circulation is limited by the narrowed blood vessel. *Marfan's syndrome* is a genetic condition in which the heart is one of the organs commonly involved.

Whatever the pathophysiology of the condition, the issue in all these defects is how well the heart is able to cope with the added demands of pregnancy and birth. Women with severe cardiac disease generally carry the highest maternal mortality risk whatever their underlying pathology

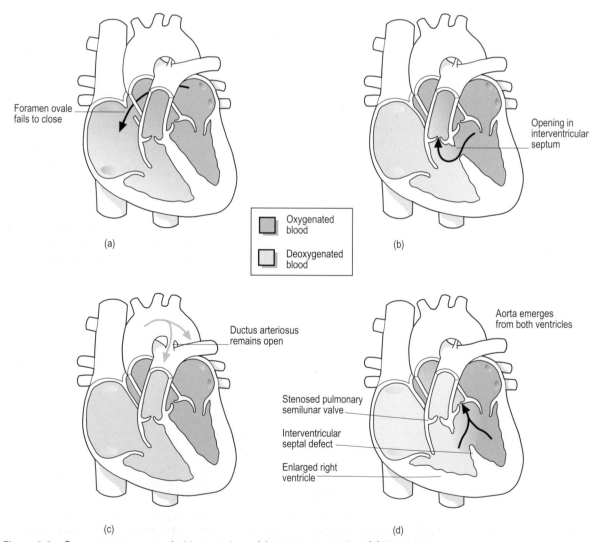

Foramen ovale fails to close

Opening in interventricular septum

Oxygenated blood

Deoxygenated blood

(a)

(b)

Ductus arteriosus remains open

Aorta emerges from both ventricles

Stenosed pulmonary semilunar valve

Interventricular septal defect

Enlarged right ventricle

(c)

(d)

Figure 3.3 Some common congenital heart defects. (a) Atrial septal defect. (b) Ventricular septal defect. (c) Patent ductus arteriosus. (d) Tetralogy of Fallot.

(Mooney 2007). The midwife must be aware of the possibility of cardiac disease and be alert for signs of a stressed heart.

Signs and symptoms

It can be difficult to identify the early signs and symptoms of cardiac disease in pregnancy, as pregnancy itself produces a similar response in the body, as discussed above. However, careful surveillance of the pregnant woman with knowledge of her baseline vital signs will alert the midwife to possible complications unrelated directly to pregnancy.

Signs and symptoms of cardiac disease include:

- Fatigue as the heart is unable to meet the needs of body cells and organs particularly on exercising

- Shortness of breath – dyspnoea – severe enough to limit normal activity, as the heart is unable to circulate blood quickly enough through the lungs to allow sufficient gaseous exchange to take place

- Palpitations due to heart arrhythmias

- Bounding, collapsing pulse as the heart rate increases without corresponding increase in cardiac output

- Chest pain associated with activity due to ischaemic heart muscle

- Peripheral oedema due to inadequate venous return.

A classification system has been developed to identify the degree of cardiac compromise based on the signs and symptoms present (Table 3.1).

Diagnosis

All women should have a physical examination in early pregnancy or preferably before conception to identify any existing problems. This may identify

---

Box 3.3 Fallot's tetralogy

Fallot's tetralogy is a congenital abnormality of the heart with four major defects: a ventricular septal defect, pulmonary stenosis, an overriding aorta and right ventricular hypertrophy. The result of these abnormalities is reduced oxygenation of blood because of movement of deoxygenated blood into the left ventricle through the VSD. This is aggravated by the presence of pulmonary stenosis. The condition is suspected when the infant develops cyanosis soon after birth or within the first few months of birth. A simple chest X-ray will identify the condition in most cases, as the heart presents with a typical boot-like shape. Treatment is by surgery.

Life-long follow-up is required as, despite improving surgical techniques, the pulmonary valve may become leaky as the heart grows and the patient may display arrhythmias due to damage to the heart's conduction system during surgery.

Table 3.1   New York classification of cardiovascular disease

Classification	Patient characteristics
Class One – No objective evidence of cardiovascular disease	Patients with cardiac disease but without resulting limitation of physical activity. Ordinary physical activity does not cause undue fatigue, palpitation, dyspnoea or angina
Class Two – Objective evidence of minimal cardiovascular disease	Patients with cardiac disease resulting in slight limitation of physical activity. They are comfortable at rest. Ordinary physical activity results in fatigue, palpitation, dyspnoea or angina
Class Three – Objective evidence of moderately severe cardiovascular disease	Patients with cardiac disease resulting in marked limitation of physical activity. They are comfortable at rest. Less than ordinary activity causes fatigue, palpitation, dyspnoea or angina
Class Four – Objective evidence of severe cardiovascular disease	Patients with cardiac disease resulting in inability to carry on any physical activity without discomfort. Symptoms of heart failure or angina may be present even at rest. If any physical activity is undertaken, discomfort increases

abnormal heart sounds indicative of heart disease. These women can be thoroughly investigated and treatment commenced before their health and the health of the fetus is compromised.

For those women who present later in pregnancy with signs of a compromised heart, diagnosis is usually based on electrocardiogram (ECG) and laboratory tests, such as blood tests, chest X-rays and echocardiography. Chest X-rays are considered safe later in pregnancy and should always be performed in women with chest pain (Lewis & Drife 2004).

Women in whom there is a known problem will be monitored closely for signs of their condition worsening.

Management of pregnancy and birth

The workload of the heart increases from early pregnancy and for the already compromised heart, there are three critical periods during the childbearing process:

1. Around 28–32 weeks' gestation is critical, as at this time, the haemodynamic changes of pregnancy reach their peak.

2. During labour is a critical period as the physical stress of uterine contractions and the psychological stress of labour pain both result in increased cardiac output.

3. From 12–24 h postpartum is critical as this is when blood from the uterus and placental bed returns to the systemic circulation.

Most women with cardiac disease can expect a good outcome from their pregnancy. The risks of a pregnancy depend on the severity of the cardiac disorder and whether the woman develops a pregnancy-related disorder. As already discussed, pregnancy brings changes to the body which put an increased workload on the heart. It depends on the severity of the cardiac disorder and the extent to which this affects function as to whether the heart is able to cope with the extra work. Any compounding disorders relating to pregnancy may precipitate heart failure and lead to maternal and/or fetal compromise. Anaemia, pre-eclampsia, haemorrhage and thrombosis are all much more serious in the woman with a cardiac defect.

Preconception care

The woman with a pre-existing cardiac disorder should be given pre-conception counselling regarding the risks to herself and her baby should she embark on a pregnancy. She will be advised to achieve optimal health before embarking on the pregnancy in order to minimize this risk. Issues such as weight, smoking, a healthy diet, rest and the prevention of anaemia can all be addressed. She can be advised to seek dental advice before pregnancy to minimize the possibility of requiring dental treatment during pregnancy, which carries a risk of endocarditis.

Pregnancy

All women with cardiac disease should be managed by a multidisciplinary team which should include the midwife, obstetrician, cardiologist and anaesthetist. These women will be seen more frequently than those with uncomplicated pregnancies. Ideally, this should be organized at a joint clinic where all team members are available, to minimize the number of visits required.

The degree to which the presence of cardiac disease complicates pregnancy depends on its severity. With adequate rest and a good diet, most women will be able to cope with pregnancy well. At each visit to the multidisciplinary team, she will be clinically examined to assess how well her heart is coping with the increasing workload of pregnancy. Fetal growth will be assessed regularly by ultrasound, and Doppler studies of placental blood flow undertaken if indicated. An anomaly scan will be offered at 16–18 weeks to check for congenital abnormality, as there is an increased risk of cardiac defect in these babies.

Diet will be assessed and adjusted, particularly if there are pharmacological considerations. Women on some diuretics will require a diet rich in potassium and low in sodium to prevent electrolyte imbalance. Prevention of anaemia is essential as lack of oxygen carrying capacity will increase the workload of the heart further.

Care will be taken to prevent infection in pregnancy. Fever will add to the load on the heart and the infective organism may precipitate or aggravate endocarditis. Should dental treatment be required, prophylactic antibiotic cover will be recommended. Ideally however, all dental work will have been carried out pre-pregnancy.

Anticoagulant therapy will be considered or reviewed. Warfarin is teratogenic and thus cannot be used in early pregnancy. It is also associated with high fetal loss in pregnancy (Lloyd 2003). Unfractionated heparin has been the anticoagulant of choice as it does not cross the placenta but can result in complications such as thrombocytopenia and osteoporosis. Subcutaneous low molecular weight heparin is now available and is recommended as it has been found to be an effective anticoagulant with minimal side-effects (see Ch. 4). Women with cardiac disease are at increased risk of developing thromboembolism, and anticoagulants should be administered throughout pregnancy (Oakley et al 2003).

Other drugs may be required throughout pregnancy. The effects of antihypertensives and antidysrhythmics on pregnancy and the developing fetus are unclear and their use needs to be balanced against possible effects (Box 3.4).

Later in pregnancy, women with a cardiac disorder may require hospitalization for rest and closer monitoring. Whenever the pregnant woman is advised to take bed rest or admitted to hospital, she should be advised to wear thromboembolic stockings.

Box 3.4 Use of digoxin in pregnancy

Digoxin is a drug used to treat cardiac failure and arrhythmias. This drug is safe to use in pregnancy providing it remains within the therapeutic range (Jordan 2002). During pregnancy, careful monitoring will ascertain whether the normal physiological changes are affecting these levels. The woman on digoxin must be advised about diet and will be advised to eat plenty of fruit, vegetables and muesli to ensure adequate levels of potassium and magnesium as deficiencies of these electrolytes in particular predispose to digoxin toxicity. Small quantities of digoxin cross the placenta and enter breast milk. However, the neonate is particularly susceptible to digoxin and although the effects are likely to be minimal, the midwife should be alert for poor weight gain.

Labour

In view of the increased risk surrounding labour, the woman with cardiac disease is advised to plan her birth in an obstetric unit where all the specialist services are available, such as neonatal intensive care and haematology. The multidisciplinary team will discuss with the woman the optimum time to give birth. Spontaneous vaginal birth is preferred to caesarean section because it causes less strain on the body. Induction of labour is not considered unless the risks of the pregnancy continuing outweigh the risks to the woman. Prostaglandins cause a dramatic increase in cardiac output while Syntocinon given by intravenous infusion results in fluid retention.

Women with cardiac disorders often have quick uncomplicated labours but it is essential that physical and psychological stress is kept to a minimum and thus the woman must be given adequate analgesia. All forms of analgesia are available to this woman. An epidural would however be the analgesic of choice, as it decreases cardiac output and causes vasodilation, reducing venous resistance (Witcher & Harvey 2006).

Throughout labour, a woman with heart disease will require very close monitoring. The use of a high dependency labour room may be useful. In addition to the normal vital signs, she may require pulse oximetry to ensure adequate oxygenation of blood for the increased workload of labour. Oxygen therapy may be required. Electrocardiography may be undertaken in women with severe heart disease (Box 3.5). Fluid balance should be monitored closely, possibly with the use of a central venous pressure (CVP) catheter.

Women with heart disease will be advised to adopt an upright or left lateral position for labour to prevent aortocaval compression (Fig. 3.4).

The second stage of labour should proceed with minimal effort by the woman. Women with cardiac disease often have a comparatively easy birth. Directed pushing must not be encouraged as this may be dangerous to the woman with a compromised heart. If birth does not proceed reasonably quickly with spontaneous pushing, a forceps delivery may be considered. A left lateral tilt is advisable to prevent aortocaval compression and care must be taken when placing the woman

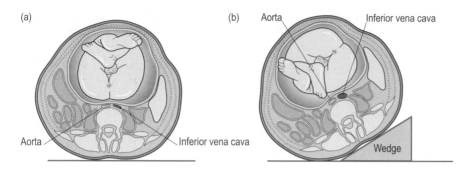

(a)

(b)

Aorta

Inferior vena cava

Aorta

Inferior vena cava

Wedge

Figure 3.4 Aortocaval compression. (a) Supine position: aorta and inferior vena cava are compressed by the fetus. (b) Left lateral tilt: uterus displacement away from aorta and vena cava.

Box 3.5 Electrocardiogram

Organized rhythmical electrical activity in the heart ensures efficient contraction of the chambers of the heart. The sinoatrial node situated in the right atrium is composed of autorhythmic cells which initiate the cardiac impulse, action potentials that spread across the heart muscle. An electrocardiogram (ECG) records electrical activity in the heart through the use of electrodes placed on the chest and limbs of the individual. Each electrode records slightly different electrical activity because of its placement on the body. A normal electrocardiogram will be displayed as a sinus wave (Fig. 3.5). The P wave records depolarization of the atria just before they contract. The QRS complex indicates ventricular depolarization and finally the T wave indicates ventricular repolarization. Any alterations in this pattern will identify heart defects. For example, a large P wave may indicate an enlarged atrium possibly due to mitral stenosis, whereas an enlarged Q wave may indicate an MI.

---

in the lithotomy position, so that there is no sudden return of blood from the legs to the heart.

Because of the added risks to the heart from loss of circulatory volume, such as occurs with haemorrhage, it is advisable to manage the third stage actively. Both Syntocinon and ergometrine have side-effects that can affect cardiac function. Ergometrine affects all smooth muscle and is absolutely contraindicated. Syntocinon is the drug of choice although it can cause hypotension and/or tachycardia, both of which put an added strain on the heart. Therefore, slow intravenous administration of this drug is advised.

Puerperium

During the first 12–24 h after birth, the heart has to cope with increased circulatory volume of fluid that has been returned from the uterine circulation. Cardiac output increases by up to 75% above pre-birth values (Dobbenga-Rhodes & Prive 2006). The woman therefore should be closely monitored for at least the first 48 h after birth to identify any signs of cardiac failure. Throughout the puerperium the heart is again at risk should any complications such as infection, fever or haemorrhage occur. Although the mother should be encouraged to rest, this increases the risk of thrombosis and thromboembolic stockings should be worn.

Cardiac arrest is rare in maternity services but the woman with a severely compromised heart may develop life-threatening complications. The multidisciplinary team will make arrangements to see these women more frequently throughout the childbearing process and she may require admission to a high dependency unit. Highly trained staff will be required to care for her and her family including midwives with training in

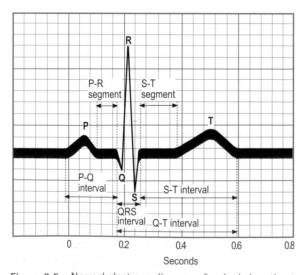

Figure 3.5 Normal electrocardiogram of a single heartbeat.

high dependency care. All members of the team will require regular updates in basic life support, and emergency drills for maternal resuscitation should be regularly practised in all obstetric units (Lewis & Drife 2004). These drills should include identification of equipment required and an examination of appropriate methods to ensure prompt arrival of a cardiac arrest team.

Midwifery management

Care of a woman with a cardiac disorder is outside the domain of the midwife (NMC 2004). Thus, any such woman who consults a midwife must be referred to the appropriate medical practitioner. A midwife will however continue to give care as part of the multidisciplinary team. Not all women are diagnosed before pregnancy however, so the midwife must be alert for any signs of cardiac compromise when examining a woman during pregnancy. Ideally, these women will have had the opportunity for preconception counselling and the midwife will have a baseline on which to compare how the body adapts to pregnancy.

As with all women, the midwife's role in pregnancy is to observe for maternal and fetal wellbeing. At each visit, the midwife will check the woman's blood pressure and urine, and thus be alerted to any indications of cardiac compromise. Promoting a well-balanced diet will benefit all women and particularly those with cardiac disorders, as this may prevent the development of anaemia. Controlling weight gain is essential to prevent even more stress on the heart and the midwife may need to refer the woman to the dietician for further advice.

One of the most important areas in which the midwife can give care is by ensuring that the woman and her family understand the management of her condition. She must encourage the woman to rest and accept help from family and friends in looking after other children. Planning care for the family and children early in pregnancy will reduce the woman's anxiety about these issues. The midwife must also ensure that the woman and her family understand fully the importance of complying with medication. Constant reassurance about all aspects of the pregnancy will hopefully minimize psychological stress.

During labour, the midwife will continue to facilitate as normal a birthing process as is feasible depending on the woman's condition. Allowing the woman to adopt a comfortable position of her choice will be encouraged, as will the involvement of her companion in the process. This will be a very frightening experience for both partners and the midwife can minimize this by giving a balanced realistic account of the likely outcome of the labour. All care will be carefully documented to ensure good teamwork.

After the birth, the woman's condition will continue to be monitored closely. This is a time of increased risk with the return of a large volume of blood from the uterine circulation into the systemic circulation. Breast-feeding and care of the baby will be encouraged and supported.

The neonate

The risks to the fetus are considerable. Pre-term birth and intrauterine growth restriction all bring added risks. Additionally, there is evidence to suggest that in the long term, the neonate with a low birthweight is at increased risk of developing ischaemic heart disease later in life (Smith et al 2001). In addition, if the mother suffers from a congenital form of cardiac disease, the infant has a 2–16% risk of presenting with congenital heart disease (Mooney 2007). In the general population, congenital heart disease occurs in only eight babies in every 1000 (McGrath 2006).

Future pregnancies

For the woman with a cardiac disease, each pregnancy carries risk. Developing a good relationship with the mother will enable the midwife to determine any future plans for more children. During the postnatal period, the midwife can then begin the process of preconception counselling and encourage careful family planning. For many women with cardiac problems, contraceptive choice is limited. The contraceptive pill is not advised as there will be a greater risk from hypertension or thromboembolism. The intrauterine contraceptive device increases the risks of infection and endocarditis. Barrier methods are a safe option but have issues of compliance. Despite this, the midwife must emphasize that planning future pregnancies is vitally important.

REFERENCES

Avila W S, Rossi E G, Ramires J A et al 2003 Pregnancy in patients with heart disease: experience with 1000 cases. Clinical Cardiology 26:135–142

Baird S M, Kennedy B 2006 Myocardial infarction in pregnancy. Journal of Perinatal & Neonatal Nursing 20(4):311–328

Dobbenga-Rhodes Y A, Prive A M 2006 Assessment and evaluation of the woman with cardiac disease during pregnancy. Journal of Perinatal & Neonatal Nursing 20(4):295–308

Foxton 2003 CHD prevention: the importance of identifying dyslipidaemia. British Journal of Nursing 12(16):950–958

Gilbert E S, Harmon J S 1998 High risk pregnancy and delivery. Mosby, St Louis

Iserin L 2001 Management of pregnancy in women with congenital heart disease. Heart 85(5):493–494

Jordan S 2002 Pharmacology for midwives. Palgrave, Houndmills, p 223–253

Lee R 2005 Thromboembolism in pregnancy: a continuing conundrum. Annals of Internal Medicine 43(10):749–750

Lewis G, Drife J (eds) 2004 Why Mothers Die 2000–2002: The sixth report of the Confidential Enquires into Maternal Deaths in the United Kingdom. RCOG, London

Lloyd C 2003 Common medical disorders associated with pregnancy. In: Fraser DM, Cooper MA (eds) Myles textbook for midwives. Churchill Livingstone, Edinburgh, p 321–355

McGrath J C 2006 Early detection and immediate management of congenital heart disease is important to long-terms outcomes. Journal of Perinatal & Neonatal Nursing 20(4):285–286

Mooney M 2007 Managing cardiac disease in pregnancy British Journal of Midwifery 15(2):76–78

Nursing and Midwifery Council 2004 Midwives rules and standards. NMC, London

Oakley C, Child A, Lung B 2003 Expert consensus document on management of cardiovascular diseases during pregnancy. European Heart Journal 24:761–781

Palmer D G 2006 Peripartum cardiomyopathy. Journal of Perinatal & Neonatal Nursing 20(4):324–334

Smith G C S, Pell J P, Walsh D 2001 Pregnancy complications and maternal risk of ischaemic heart disease: a retrospective cohort study of 129,290 births. Lancet 357(9273):2002–2006

Swinburne C 2004 Take heart. Nursing Standard 18(42):18–19

Witcher P M, Harvey C J 2006 Modifying labor routines for the woman with cardiac disease. Journal of Perinatal & Neonatal Nursing 20(4):303–311

Chapter 4

Thromboembolic disorders

INTRODUCTION

Thromboembolic disorders are the leading cause of direct maternal death in the UK (Lewis & Drife 2004).

From 2000–2002, 30 women died from thrombosis and/or embolism in the UK. Some 25 deaths were as a result of a pulmonary embolism and five from cerebral vein thrombosis. Of the deaths from pulmonary embolism, four deaths occurred in pregnancy, one in labour and 17 postnatally. Some 16 of these women had risk factors for thromboembolic disorders. In 57% of all cases, there was evidence of substandard care. Prophylactic anticoagulants are strongly recommended in all areas of healthcare where mobility is limited and this must be a consideration in the care of women undergoing childbirth dependent on risk (RCOG 2004). The majority of thromboembolic events during the childbearing process are not fatal, but may be responsible for considerable long-term morbidity (Gates 2000).

The midwife is the leading care giver in the majority of pregnancies and as such must be fully aware of all risk factors that may lead to a negative outcome. It is essential therefore, that she has a thorough understanding of thromboembolic disorders and their treatment in order to recognize those at risk and ensure prompt referral and treatment.

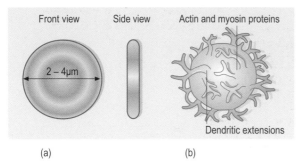

Figure 4.1   Diagrammatic representation of a platelet. (a) Inactive platelet. (b) Activated platelet.

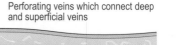
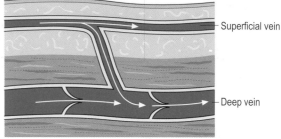

Figure 4.2   Veins of the lower limb.

RELEVANT ANATOMY AND PHYSIOLOGY

The control and role of blood pressure in the movement of blood through the circulatory system has already been explained (see Ch. 2). The continued brisk movement of blood through blood vessels is one of the factors that prevents coagulation and thrombosis. Control of the coagulation cascade is another.

The circulating fluid in the cardiovascular system, blood, is composed of two main elements. Plasma is a fluid and blood cells are suspended within this.

Plasma is a straw coloured substance similar in composition to interstitial fluid. It makes up approximately 55% of the blood volume and is essential for the maintenance of homeostasis. Plasma is composed of 90% water plus dissolved or suspended substances. These include nutrients, wastes, proteins and the products of cell metabolism. Chemicals and proteins involved in the coagulation of blood are transported in this way.

The remaining 45% of blood is composed of blood cells:

- Erythrocytes – red blood cells – are responsible for transporting oxygen from the lungs to all parts of the body; 99% of blood cells are erythrocytes
- Leucocytes – white blood cells – make up approximately 1% of blood cells and are involved in infection control and the inflammatory response
- Thrombocytes – platelets – are very small fragments of cellular material. These contain the substances essential to blood clotting (Fig. 4.1a,b).

Movement of blood through the circulation is controlled primarily by contraction of the heart.

Blood pressure exerted by this process and by the constraining influence of the walls of the blood vessels moves blood rapidly through the arterial network. Blood pressure gradually drops as blood vessels become narrower, and once blood has passed through the capillary network, pressure is comparatively low. Additionally gravity plays a role (see Ch. 2). Venous return of blood to the heart is therefore more easily disrupted and it is in the venous system that there is increased risk of the formation of a thrombus particularly in lower limbs.

The venous system of the lower limbs consists of three distinct types of vein; deep veins which lie within the skeletal muscles (femoral, tibial and popliteal); superficial veins which lie outside this sheath (long and short saphenous veins); and joining the two systems, perforating or communicating veins (Fig. 4.2).

Venous circulation in lower limbs returns blood to the heart in an upward direction against the force of gravity. This upward flow is maintained by valves which prevent backflow.

Valves are folds of the tunica intima which lines the veins (Fig. 4.3). The tunica intima is a very thin layer consisting of the basement membrane and endothelium. Valves can thus be easily damaged by injury to the blood vessels. In some individuals, valves are inherently incompetent and the upward flow is more difficult to maintain.

Venous return depends therefore on several factors:

- Difference in blood pressure between venules, approximately 16 mmHg, and the right atrium, 0 mmHg. Although this is a comparatively small pressure differential, resistance in veins is

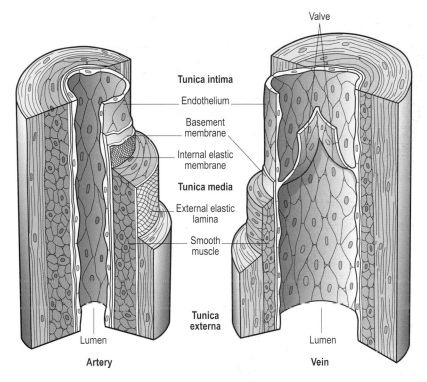

Figure 4.3   Comparison of the anatomy of an artery and a vein.

Tunica intima
Endothelium
Basement membrane
Internal elastic membrane
Tunica media
External elastic lamina
Smooth muscle
Tunica externa
Valve
Lumen
Lumen
Artery
Vein

very low. Additionally, as the right atrium empties with each contraction of the heart, blood is sucked into the vacuum that is left

- Skeletal muscle contractions: Deep veins running through skeletal muscle are squeezed by muscle contraction and raise blood pressure. Blood is forced along the veins in the direction of the heart and backflow is prevented by the presence of the valves. When the muscles relax, the valves close and prevent backflow (Fig. 4.4). Normal daily activities require regular skeletal muscular contraction during walking, working etc. and thus contribute to this process
- Respiration: During inspiration, the diaphragm moves downward. This results in a decrease in pressure in the thorax and an increase in the abdominal cavity. As a result, blood moves from compressed abdominal veins into decompressed thoracic veins. During expiration, the presence of valves in veins again prevents backflow.

Haemostasis (cessation of bleeding)

Blood is essential to life. It is imperative that any loss of this substance due to trauma of a blood

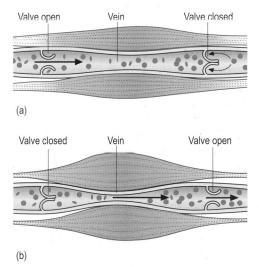

Valve open   Vein   Valve closed

(a)

Valve closed   Vein   Valve open

(b)

Figure 4.4   Movement of blood by skeletal muscle contraction. (a) Relaxed skeletal muscle. (b) Contracting skeletal muscle.

vessel is corrected as quickly as possible. The body has a range of measures it can bring into play to seal the blood vessel and minimize blood loss (Fig. 4.5).

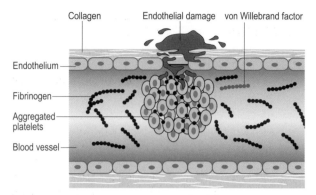

Figure 4.5   Haemostasis.

Initially, on detecting a damaged blood vessel, thrombocytes release serotonin which, along with other chemicals released by the damaged cells, causes local vasoconstriction of the blood vessel to minimize blood loss. Around the site of the trauma, thrombocytes clump together and release substances such as ADP, which attract many more platelets to the area, adding to the size of the temporary plug formed (Walthall 2006). Coagulation of blood occurs around the plug forming a permanent clot.

Coagulation is a complex process involving two pathways and a series of steps in each (Fig. 4.6). In summary, strands of fibrin are synthesized by a plasma protein, fibrinogen, which combines with water and solutes to form a gel in which blood cells become trapped. This is the thrombus – blood clot. As further chemicals become involved, the thrombus hardens and seals the blood vessel, and also acts as scaffolding for the repair of the damaged blood vessel. Finally, on completion of the repair, the fibrin thrombus is dissolved by the process of fibrinolysis to re-open the blood vessel fully for effective blood flow.

In undamaged blood vessels, various anti-clotting mechanisms restrict and prevent clot formation. Normal blood flow depends on a delicate balance between circulating and endothelial anticoagulant and procoagulating factors. It is when this fine balance is disrupted that an inappropriate thrombus forms. The hormonal changes of pregnancy disrupt this balance to some extent in all women; in women with an additional risk factor, this may result in the production of a thrombus.

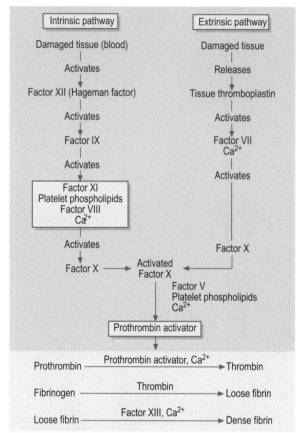

Figure 4.6   The coagulation cascade.

PATHOPHYSIOLOGY OF THROMBOEMBOLISM

Any situation in which blood flow is slow or disrupted places the individual at risk of a thromboembolic event. Recent press has highlighted this risk in publicizing the dangers of immobility aggravated by dehydration on 'long haul' flights (Box 4.1). This risk has been well recognized for many years in healthcare and has led to rapid mobilization and physiotherapy in all patients post-surgery. Despite this, thromboembolic disorders continue to result in high mortality and morbidity rates, with commensurate healthcare costs.

Aetiology

A thrombosis is the formation of a clot – thrombus – inside a blood vessel, thus obstructing the flow of

Box 4.1 DVT and long haul flying

Pathophysiological changes associated with flying give rise to several significant predisposing factors for developing a DVT (Shepherd & Edwards 2004). Hypoxia and vasoconstriction develop over time and at high altitudes due to an increase in blood pressure and heart rate. Cabin pressure is set for 6000 feet and long haul flights take place at much higher levels. These changes are aggravated by immobility and dehydration. After 1 h at these high altitudes, there is a decrease in blood flow to the lower limbs and pooling of plasma proteins (Willcox 2004), thus increasing the risk of thrombosis. Additionally, pressure from the seat on the back of the leg and the cramped conditions in economy seats increase the risk factors. Antiembolic stockings can be considered to reduce this risk but these are not suitable for some people with pre-existing disease (Scurr et al 2001). Walking around the aisles of the aircraft and preventing dehydration by drinking water (not alcohol) will help reduce the risks of DVT.

removal of fluid. Common causes of venous stasis are (Gutierrez & Peterson 2002):

- A sedentary lifestyle
- Compression of blood vessels as in obesity or an abdominal tumour
- Congestive heart failure
- Chronic venous disease.

There are two main types of thrombus – venous and arterial. Venous thrombosis can occur in any of the veins of the body, for example a deep venous thrombosis. Common arterial thromboses are found in the coronary arteries, resulting in a myocardial infarction, or in cerebral arteries, causing a cerebrovascular accident ('stroke'). Both of these disorders can also be caused by an embolism, but a myocardial infarction is often the result of damage to the blood vessel walls by atherosclerotic plaque to which platelets are attracted. A cerebrovascular accident (CVA) can have many causes including thrombosis due atherosclerosis (see Ch. 8).

Thromboembolic related conditions

Varicose veins

Blood flow in legs can slow and pool during inactivity of skeletal muscle. This is particularly true for those whose occupations require them to stand for long periods (Bentley 2003). When the plantar veins are compressed, as in walking, blood flow is increased into deep veins. Pressure in the veins is highest on standing but decreases on walking. In the supine position, blood pressure in the veins is negligible.

Varicose veins, or varicosities, are veins in which blood flow has become sluggish on its return to the heart, usually as a result of increased resistance. The valves in the veins are weak and incompetent and allow backflow, and as a result, the vessel walls become dilated and tortuous. Superficial and perforating veins, unsupported by skeletal muscle, are particularly susceptible. This aggravates venous stasis and predisposes to the formation of a thrombus. Although increased resistance leads to the development of varicose veins, there is a strong familial tendency to have inherently weak vessel walls.

blood through the circulatory system. The term 'thromboembolism' is a term applied to the formation of a thrombus complicated by the risk of embolization. An embolus is a moving clot.

Classically, the development of an inappropriate thrombosis is caused by a disruption in one or more of the following (Virchow's triad 1856):

- Alteration of blood flow (haemostasis)
- Injury of the vascular endothelium
- Alterations to the constitution of the blood (hypercoagulability).

Commonly, the formation of the thrombus is caused by an injury to the blood vessel wall, either by trauma or infection, or by slowing or stagnation of blood flow past this injury. Abnormalities in the coagulation process may aggravate or initiate this process.

Alternatively and frequently the issue in caring for those in hospital, the formation of a thrombus is initiated in the first instance by venous stasis.

Venous stasis describes any condition in which venous blood flow slows or stagnates and occurs as a result of an overabundance of, or decreased

Common sites for varicosities are:

- In the legs where the body's upright stance and the effect of gravity slow blood flow
- In the anal canal, haemorrhoids
- In vulvar veins in pregnant women due to pressure from the enlarging uterus.

The presence of varicose veins is commonly indicated by localized swelling, which on examination can be felt, and subsequently seen, as being the result of swollen and knotty superficial veins. The patient complains of heavy, aching legs. Discolouration is seen due to the accumulation of waste products and dry itchy skin develops over the varicose vein. The veins readily become inflamed – phlebitis – and occasionally the vessel wall ruptures causing haemorrhage. Feet and ankles may become swollen and symptoms increase during the course of the day, particularly if the woman has been standing for a long time.

Diagnosis is determined by the *Trendelenburg test*. In this procedure, the leg is elevated from a horizontal position to empty the veins, and on standing, the veins are observed as they refill. Normally filling is comparatively slow: in the presence of varicosities, filling is much more rapid as the incompetent valves allow filling from above as well as below. Doppler studies will confirm the structure and functioning of the veins.

Medical management involves the use of support stockings and advice to avoid prolonged standing. Elevation of the limb will assist drainage and can be achieved by raising the foot of the bed at night. However, surgical treatment is often required. Affected veins are ligated and stripped, encouraging blood to return to the heart via the deep veins of the leg.

Haemorrhoids are varicosities of the anus and rectum. These can occur both at the anal margin and in the rectum. Haemorrhoids are a common complaint and occur as a result of inherently weak vessel walls combined with other factors, such as constipation and pregnancy.

Deep vein thrombosis

A deep vein thrombosis (DVT) is an aggregation of blood cells and platelets trapped within a meshwork of fibrin, which causes obstruction in a vein (Wilmott & Alikhan 2002). The vein affected is usually one of the deep veins of the lower limb, although clots can also develop in the pelvic and upper veins of the body.

A DVT is usually caused by venous stasis as a result of one of the following factors (Walsh 2002):

- Varicose veins
- Over 40 years of age
- Clinical history/family history of DVT or pulmonary embolism
- Immobility due to prolonged bed rest
- Surgery lasting longer than 30 min
- Pregnancy
- Serious illness such as infection, myocardial infarction
- Abnormal clotting disorders (Box 4.2)
- Obesity
- Malignancy
- Thrombophilia
- Economy class syndrome – long haul flights in cramped conditions.

Box 4.2 Haemophilia

Haemophilia is an X-linked recessive genetic condition in which there is impaired coagulation of the blood. In 80% of people with haemophilia, there is a deficiency of clotting factor VIII. Another 20% of people have a deficiency in clotting factor IX – Christmas disease.

As this is a sex-linked trait, the condition is transmitted through the female line to their male offspring. As the female has a second X chromosome, she is therefore a carrier of the condition. The male however will suffer overtly from the condition.

Haemophilia is a debilitating and crippling disorder that seriously endangers the sufferer's life. When a blood vessel is injured, the normal clot and scab forming process does not happen and the blood vessel continues to bleed for a long time. Bleeding can be external as in a cut or internal into muscles, joints or organs. In the latter, the sufferer will experience pain as a first warning that internal bleeding is taking place.

The individual requires regular injections of the missing factor and has to learn to avoid trauma and obtain prompt treatment for bleeding episodes.

Haemophilia figured prominently in Queen Victoria's family. She passed the genetic mutation through her daughters down a long line of royals across Europe.

A DVT may be asymptomatic and is difficult to diagnose by physical examination. One of the most effective methods of decreasing mortality and morbidity rates from a thromboembolic disorder is therefore to recognize those at risk and consider prophylactic measures such as TED stockings and anticoagulant therapy. *Thromboprophylaxis* is the process involved in preventing the formation of a clot.

Thromboprophylaxis can be mechanical or pharmacological:

- *Mechanical methods* include the application of antiembolic stockings, which act primarily by altering blood flow. Antiembolic stockings inhibit two of the factors identified in Virchow's triad – damage to the blood vessel and stasis (Cock 2006). They work by applying external pressure to the vein, resulting in the cusps of the valves meeting in the midline, improving the rate of blood flow and reducing venous hypertension. Stockings must be medically prescribed and carefully fitted to size

- *Pharmacological prophylaxis* involves the use of heparin-based compounds and alters the activity of the enzymes involved in the normal clotting process.

Signs and symptoms of deep vein thrombosis are not always present but include pain in the calf area, especially on walking, with localized tenderness. Swelling and increased skin temperature may occur around the site of the thrombosis. Erythema may be present and surface veins may become dilated. Pitting oedema may be present. Measurement of the affected leg may show a disparity with that of the unaffected leg.

Diagnosis Ultrasound Doppler studies may demonstrate this condition (Eagle 2006) but often diagnosis is based on the present of risk factors and complicating features.

Treatment Treatment is aimed at identifying and treating the cause. Anticoagulant therapy is initiated as soon as a diagnosis is made. This is commonly via a bolus dose of heparin followed by either an intravenous infusion of heparin, or subcutaneous low molecular weight heparin. Adequate anticoagulation is determined by regular measurement of APTT (activated partial thromboplastin time). Heparin acts by preventing further clot formation. An oral anticoagulant is also commenced but takes around 3 days to prolong the prothrombin time adequately to be used as first line treatment (Walsh 2002).

Elevation and movement are the simplest methods to reduce the oedema associated with this condition. Compression stockings should be used where increased activity or immediate treatment of the cause is not possible. These act by counteracting the increased pressure in the capillary bed, thus reducing venous pooling and oedema.

Prognosis When identified early and treated appropriately, prognosis is good. The danger arises due to the risk of a section of the thrombus breaking free, and travelling within the circulation as an embolism. This may lead to the embolus lodging in the smaller blood vessels of the body particularly those of the lungs. It must be appreciated that the blood vessels leading away from the veins of the legs increase in diameter; blood then passes through the heart and goes to the pulmonary circulation, through vessels that are now decreasing in diameter. Thus, the pulmonary vasculature is the most likely site for the embolus to lodge, forming a pulmonary embolism, a life-threatening condition.

Thrombophlebitis and phlebothrombosis

Phlebitis is an inflammation of the walls of a vein as a result of injury or infection. Circulating platelets detect the damage and initiate the coagulation cascade to form a clot around the injury – a condition known as thrombophlebitis. Phlebothrombosis is the formation of a clot within a vein with no associated inflammation often due to venous stasis as in prolonged bed rest. Again, the risks in these conditions is the thrombosis which has the potential to throw off emboli or indeed be carried along in the blood as an embolism itself.

The signs and symptoms of thrombophlebitis are localized pain with tenderness and swelling. The pain can be quite severe. In superficial veins, the skin may be reddened and warm to the touch. If a leg is involved, calf pain may be produced during dorsiflexion. Other symptoms include fever and general malaise.

Treatment   Thrombophlebitis normally subsides quite quickly. Non-steroidal anti-inflammatory drugs will ease the pain and reduce swelling.

Pulmonary embolism

A pulmonary embolism (PE) is *common, deadly and frequently unsuspected* (Reid 1999). A PE is a blockage in one of the arteries of the lungs by a blood clot, or other substance such as air or fat. The most common cause of a pulmonary embolism is blockage from an embolus that has been dislodged from the femoral or iliac veins. Emboli break off for a variety of reasons including trauma or increased venous pressure. Once free, the embolus migrates up the vena cava, through the right atrium and ventricle of the heart and into the narrowing pulmonary arteries.

The pathophysiological effects depend on the size of the embolus. Small to moderate emboli may cause infarction of pulmonary tissue, thus preventing inflation of local alveoli. Larger emboli impede blood flow and additionally cause back pressure, reducing blood flow through the heart and impeding cardiac output. This will quickly lead to hypotension, heart failure and death.

Signs and symptoms of a pulmonary embolus are:

- Dyspnoea of sudden onset
- Tachypnoea
- Chest pain
- Cough
- Haemoptysis.

In severe cases, the patient will show signs of cyanosis, tachycardia, hypotension, shock and collapse. This is a very serious condition with a poor prognosis in many cases. Objective diagnosis is difficult however, as signs and symptoms vary considerably in severity and may indicate other pulmonary conditions. Diagnosis is therefore based on history and the exclusion of other causes by undertaking chest X-ray and electrocardiogram (ECG). Ultrasound and Doppler studies (Box 4.3) may confirm the presence of a DVT in the lower limbs, which will lead to a probable diagnosis of PE. CT scan or pulmonary angiogram, or a combination of the two may be useful in confirming the diagnosis.

Treatment is with oxygen and analgesia to prevent further deterioration of the condition.

Box 4.3 Doppler ultrasound

Ultrasound is a term applied to very high frequency sounds outside the normal hearing range. In 1842, Christian Doppler identified that the frequency of sound emitted or reflected from a moving object varied with the velocity of the object. The hand-held Doppler ultrasound uses a transducer – probe – in which ultrasonic waves are generated, to direct and detect movement of blood in blood vessels.

The Doppler ultrasound is designed to ignore reflection of sound from non-moving tissues but to amplify sound back from moving tissues particularly red blood cells (Eagle 2006). Also, the sound returning from the blood varies with the speed and direction. Thus, arterial blood will have a higher pitched sound than that generated by blood in veins. As blood moves forwards and backwards, there will be corresponding increases and decreases in pitch and loudness.

In large elastic arteries, as the blood is moved by contraction of the heart, the vessels stretch. As the heart relaxes, the arteries also relax, causing some blood to flow backwards for a short period of time. A triphasic flow is one in which there is evidence of a forwards, backwards, forwards flow – this is a normal finding. Biphasic flow indicates a forward, backwards flow and indicates a diseased and/or blocked artery.

Anticoagulant therapy is commenced initially by intravenous infusion and continued orally as described above. Thrombolysis may be considered in an attempt to dissolve the clot but this is still debatable because of the risk of bleeding. If prescribed, this may be in the form of streptokinase 250 000 units i.v. over 1 h, followed by 100 000 units i.v. per hour for 24 h. The infusion may be continued to 72 h if there is a concurrent DVT. Surgical management may be considered, although this is associated with a poor outcome in an acute pulmonary embolism.

Prognosis is often poor and depends on the amount of lung affected and the overall health of the individual.

Disseminated intravascular coagulation

Disseminated intravascular coagulation (DIC) is a condition in which disseminated (widespread) intravascular (within blood vessels) coagulation (clotting) occurs inappropriately. Chemicals from a primary disease process initiate the coagulation process leading to the production of microthrombi throughout the circulation system. This process depletes the body of platelets and coagulation factors and thus increases the risk of haemorrhage when injury to blood vessels occurs.

Disseminated intravascular coagulation usually occurs in critically ill patients secondary to conditions such as:

- Sepsis (particularly with Gram negative bacteria)
- Trauma such as surgery, burns or shock
- Cancer
- Liver disease
- Incompatible blood transfusions
- Obstetric conditions such as placental abruption (see later).

Signs and symptoms of DIC include signs of inappropriate blood loss. Bleeding from the nose or mouth, or oozing around a venepuncture site are typical signs of a coagulation disorder. Other signs may include haematuria and/or intracranial haemorrhage.

Diagnosis is based on the presence of fibrin degradation products (FDPs). DIC triggers fibrinolysis, which breaks down the fibrin in clots, the end-products of which are FDPs. FDPs further disrupt the process of coagulation and are thus good indicators of the presence of DIC.

Treatment involves replacing blood cells and coagulation factors that have been destroyed by this condition. This is usually undertaken with intravenous infusions of platelets and fresh frozen plasma.

Disseminated intravascular coagulation is associated with a poor outcome in many cases and thus identification of risk factors is essential to prevent the condition occurring. Early detection of signs of a clotting defect should be an integral component of care.

THROMBOEMBOLIC DISORDERS IN PREGNANCY

Introduction

Women are ten times more likely to develop a thrombosis during pregnancy compared with non-pregnant women of the same age (RCOG 2004).

Postnatally, the risks of developing a thromboembolic disorder are also high. Many factors are

Table 4.1 Risk factors for venous thromboembolism in pregnancy and the puerperium

Pre-existing factors	New onset or transient
• Previous thromboembolism	• Surgery
• Thrombophilia	• Hyperemesis
• Congenital coagulation defect	• Dehydration
• Antiphospholipid syndrome	• Severe infection,
• Age >35 years	e.g. pyelonephritis
• BMI >30	• Immobility
• Parity >4	• Pre-eclampsia
• Gross varicose veins	• Excessive blood
• Paraplegia	loss
• Sickle cell disease	• Long haul travel
• Inflammatory disorders, e.g. IBD	• Prolonged labour
• Medical disorders,	• Instrumental
e.g. nephritic syndrome	delivery
• Myeloproliferative disorders, e.g. essential thrombocytopenia	

associated with an increased risk of developing a thromboembolic disorder during the childbearing process (Table 4.1). It is essential therefore, that women at risk are identified early in the childbearing process and advised and treated accordingly.

Thromboembolic disorders are the leading cause of maternal death and women who have had a caesarean section are at increased risk of developing thromboembolic disease (NICE 2004). The numbers of deaths following caesarean section have however fallen over recent years but there has been no improvement in the small number of deaths that occur prenatally or postnatally in women who have experienced a vaginal birth (Lewis & Drife 2004). Of the 30 maternal deaths, 25 had risk factors for thromboembolic disorders – 13 were overweight, five had had a period of bed rest, four had a family history of thromboembolism, two had been on a long haul flight and one had varicose veins. Midwives must therefore be vigilant for risk factors and manage care of a pregnant woman in a way that does not further put the woman at risk.

Physiological changes in pregnancy

Circulatory changes in pregnancy result in an increased blood supply and expansion of the venous circulation. These changes exacerbate varicosities which predispose to thrombosis. The hormones of pregnancy aggravate this and pregnancy is commonly the time when varicose veins first appear leading to considerable discomfort.

The physiological changes of pregnancy result in an increase of 30% in venous stasis by the 15th week of pregnancy and an increase of 60% by 36 weeks (Yu et al 2006). Pregnancy is also a time of hypercoagulability. Hormonal changes and preparation for the homeostatic challenges of the third stage of labour increase the risks of developing a thrombosis particularly in those at risk. Considering Virchow's triad (1856), the factors that influence these changes are (Fig. 4.6):

- Hypercoagulability
  - Fibrinogen increases from 12 weeks by 50%
  - A slight increase in prothrombin levels
  - An increase in factors 7,8,9 & 10
  - An increase in platelets
  - A decrease in coagulation time from 12 to 8 min
- Haemostasis
  - Venous return from lower limbs is reduced due to the pregnant uterus compressing the inferior vena cava
  - Progesterone acts on the smooth muscle of blood vessels reducing tone
  - Incompetent valves in the lower limbs may further contribute to decreased blood flow
  - Right iliac vein crosses the left iliac artery decreasing blood flow still further in the left leg
- Vascular damage
  - Increased venous distension and stasis may lead to microscopic tears in blood vessels
  - Trauma may occur as a result of birth.

Incidence

Accurate data for the incidence of DVT or pulmonary embolism is difficult to achieve as many deep vein thromboses go undetected. A large study in North West Thames recently identified the prevalence of thromboembolism as 0.04% in pregnant women of normal weight compared with a risk of 0.08% in obese women (Sebire et al 2001). The majority of pulmonary emboli occur postnatally however. Over 80% of thromboembolic events

occur in the left leg as a result of the anatomical arrangement of the right and left iliac veins.

Prevention

An early history taking is essential in the prevention of thromboembolic episodes during the childbearing process, as coagulation changes occur from early in pregnancy. Preconception advice would be invaluable in identifying and in some cases, such as obesity, dealing with them before pregnancy.

Women with a previous thromboembolic event should have a detailed history taken and undergo screening for both inherited and acquired thrombophilia, before embarking on pregnancy.

Prenatally

The midwife should take a full history at an early appointment in order to recognize those at risk. Risk factors are shown in Table 4.1. Advice can then be given about maintaining a healthy lifestyle both for maternal and fetal benefit and in order to reduce risks of the development of a thrombosis. Regular exercise, smoking cessation and drinking plenty of water will all reduce risk.

The midwife will undertake a full physical examination to rule out any predisposing factors, such as varicose veins. If the woman complains of pain in her legs, the use of support tights may reduce this. If for any reason mobility is reduced, the medical team may consider prophylactic treatment such as the use of antiembolic stockings.

The presence of risk factors will indicate a need to consider pharmacological thromboprophylaxis. Evidence suggests that it is difficult to determine whether prophylaxis is beneficial in women with one of the risk factors but those with three or more risk factors should be started on low molecular weight heparin (LMWH) from early in pregnancy and for 5 days postpartum. A low molecular weight heparin (LMWH) such as enoxaparin or dalteparin given subcutaneously may be prescribed. However, this decision should be made for each individual woman depending on the severity of the risk factors especially if mobility is restricted for any reason.

Heparin is the anticoagulant of choice as the molecules are too large to cross the placental barrier;

warfarin is associated with up to 5% risk of congenital abnormalities, particularly between 6 and 12 weeks' gestation (Chan et al 2000). Warfarin also increases the risks of spontaneous abortion, fetal and maternal haemorrhage, neurological problems in the baby and stillbirth (Jordan 2002). Heparin does however have side-effects, such as thrombocytopenia, osteoporosis and allergic reactions. Low molecular weight heparins, however, are associated with fewer complications (Gates 2000).

Labour

The woman who is having pharmacological thromboprophylaxis should be advised to discontinue this at least 12h before labour commences if at all possible because of the risk of postpartum haemorrhage during the third stage (Mazlovitz et al 2005). Once admitted in labour, she will be reassessed and further doses prescribed by medical staff (RCOG 2004). All women with risk factors for thromboembolism should be advised to give birth in an obstetric unit where the multidisciplinary team can monitor closely.

During labour, care must be taken to reduce risk of thrombosis by encouraging mobility and avoiding exhaustion and dehydration. During invasive procedures, care must be taken to prevent trauma to legs, for example while using the stirrups. This is particularly important if the woman is sedated, unconscious or has no feeling in her legs during an epidural or spinal anaesthesia. In high risk women, the use of antiembolic stockings may be advised.

All women undergoing a caesarean section will be given prophylactic LMWH, which will continue until 5 days postoperatively. Coagulation studies should identify a normal haemostasis before commencing prophylaxis however. These women should also be prescribed antiembolic stockings with early mobilization and adequate hydration postoperatively.

Puerperium

In all women at risk of thromboembolism, antiembolic stockings will be advised, and prophylactic anticoagulants commenced immediately following birth provided there is no risk of haemorrhage

(RCOG 2004). In women who have had epidural or spinal anaesthesia, this will be commenced 4h after the insertion or removal of the catheter. The epidural cannula should not be removed within 12h of the most recent injection of LMWH. Women at high risk of postpartum haemorrhage may be more conveniently managed with unfractionated heparin, as this has a shorter half-life than LMWH and is more easily reversed with the administration of protamine sulphate.

As coagulation does not return to normal for several weeks after birth, thromboprophylaxis should be continued for 6 weeks in high risk women. For those at lower risk, postpartum prophylaxis of 3–5 days is sufficient. Mobility will be encouraged and in those women at high risk or with reduced mobility, leg exercises will be initiated.

During the postnatal period, the midwife will examine all women for signs of thromboembolism. However, with increasing numbers of women receiving reduced postnatal care (Anderson 2000), an essential role of the midwife is to educate women of the risk of developing a thromboembolic disorder, especially in those with an increased risk such as women with pre-eclampsia (Walraven et al 2003). Many women are not aware of these risks and do not appreciated why midwives examine legs postnatally (Reynolds 2004).

Women with varicose veins will be advised to wear support stockings and to put them on before getting out of bed in the morning. Pain or swelling in the calf may indicate thrombophlebitis or deep vein thrombosis and if present should be referred to the medical team immediately. Treatment will be commenced as described earlier. Women started on warfarin must be advised not to take other drugs without consulting their GP, as many drugs interact with warfarin, either by enhancing or reducing its anticoagulant effect (Reid 1999). The importance of taking the drug regularly at a particular time of day should also be emphasized and the woman educated about the signs of over anticoagulation, such as bleeding gums or haematuria. Warning signs of intracranial haemorrhage, such as prolonged headache or confusion are a comparatively common cause of morbidity or mortality in patients on anticoagulation. All women on anticoagulants should carry a card indicating that they are on thromboprophylaxis.

The midwife must be alert at all times for risk factors that may predispose to a pulmonary embolism and if the woman complains of chest pain and a cough, or breathlessness, a pulmonary embolism must be suspected. Urgent referral must be made to the medical team as the woman may collapse without warning.

The combined oral contraceptive pill should not be prescribed during the first 3 months after birth in women with any risk factors for thromboembolism.

Pulmonary embolism

Treatment for a suspected pulmonary embolism will be commenced even if diagnosis is uncertain (RCOG 2004). The woman will be admitted to a high dependency unit where heparin will be administered by intravenous infusion. Antiembolic stockings will be applied and she will be closely monitored. Mobility will be restricted to prevent further detachment of an embolism until diagnosis is confirmed. Heparin dosage must be closely monitored because of the risk of postpartum haemorrhage.

Management and treatment of collapse due to pulmonary embolism

This is an *obstetric emergency*. Urgent medical aid must be summoned and must include a consultant obstetrician, senior anaesthetist and a physician. The woman must be helped into the most comfortable position for breathing and oxygen administered at 8 L/min. Emergency equipment will be on hand and an intravenous infusion commenced. An ECG monitor will be attached and vital signs monitored including pulse oximetry. Pain will be relieved by a strong analgesic such as morphine to reduce shock and anticoagulant therapy commenced.

Heparin (5000 IU) will be given by bolus injection over 5 min. An intravenous infusion administering 20 IU/kg per hour will be initiated. The APPT levels will be measured after 6 h and the infusion rate of heparin adjusted accordingly. Thrombolytic agents may be administered and results are usually good if administered within the first 12 h. Careful monitoring should be undertaken to ensure that this traumatic event has not triggered DIC.

Role of the midwife in the care of a woman with a pulmonary embolism

The midwife's responsibility is to monitor the woman's condition including vital signs, fluid and electrolyte balance and recording prescribed drugs. Additionally, the midwife must attend to the emotional needs of the woman and her family and assist them in the care of their baby.

The risk of developing a thromboembolism continues well into the puerperium. This risk must be considered and treated with thromboprophylaxis in any further episode of surgery, severe infection and indeed when travelling on a long haul journey (RCOG 2004).

Neonatal considerations

Thromboembolic disorders can be either inherited or acquired. The baby of a mother who has had a thrombosis due to a genetically inherited condition may need to be carefully observed for haemorrhagic disease of the newborn.

Future pregnancies

Women with a history of a thromboembolic event have an increased risk in pregnancy (Pabinger et al 2002). Before contemplating further pregnancies, these women should undergo screening for both inherited and acquired thrombophilia, as these conditions increase the risk of thromboembolism in pregnancy and childbirth.

REFERENCES

Anderson T 2000 The state of midwifery across England. MIDIRS Midwifery Digest 10(2):385–387

Bentley J 2003 Compression therapy; how to make it effective. Practice Nursing 14(11):501–506

Chan W S, Anand S, Gusberg J S 2000 Anticoagulation of pregnant women with mechanical heart valves: a systematic review of the literature. Archives of Internal Medicine 160:191–196

Cock K A 2006 Anti-embolism stockings: are they used effectively and correctly? British Journal of Nursing 15(6): S4–S12

Eagle M 2006 Doppler ultrasound – basics revisited. British Journal of Nursing 15(11):S24–S30

Gates S 2000 Thromboembolic disease in pregnancy. Current Opinion in Obstetrics and Gynecology 12:117–122

Gutierrez K J, Peterson P G 2002 Pathophysiology. WB Saunders, Philadelphia, p 105–110

Jordan S 2002 Pharmacology for Midwives. Palgrave, Houndmills

Lewis G, Drife J (eds) 2004 Why Mothers Die 2000–2002: The sixth report of the Confidential Enquires into Maternal Deaths in the United Kingdom. RCOG, London

Mazlovitz S, Many A, Landsberg J A et al 2005 The safety of low molecular weight heparin therapy during labour Journal of Maternal-Fetal and Neonatal Medicine 17(1):39–43

National Institute for Clinical Excellence 2004 Caesarean Section Clinical Guideline 13. Online. Available at: http://www.nice.org.uk/CG013NICEguideline (accessed April 2007)

Pabinger I, Grafenhoffer H, Kyrle P A et al 2002 Temporary increase in the risk for recurrence during pregnancy in women with a history of venous thromboembolism Blood 100:1060–1062

Reid E 1999 Pulmonary embolism: an overview of treatment and nursing issues. British Journal of Nursing 8(20):1373–1378

Reynolds S I 2004 Deep vein thrombosis; are postnatal women aware? British Journal of Midwifery 12(10):636–640

Royal College of Obstetrics and Gynaecology 2004 Thromboprophylaxis during pregnancy, labour and after vaginal delivery. Guideline No. 37. RCOG, London

Scurr J H, Machin S J, Bailey-King S, McDonald S, Smith P D 2001 Frequency and prevention of symptomless deep vein thrombosis in long haul flights: A randomised controlled trial. Lancet 357(9267):1485–1489

Sebire N J, Jolly M, Harris J P et al 2001 Maternal obesity and pregnancy outcome: a study of 287,213 pregnancies in London. International Journal of Obesity Related Metabolic Disorders 25:1175–1182

Shepherd L, Edwards S L 2004 The effects of flying; processes, consequences and prevention. British Journal of Nursing 13(1):19–29

Virchow R 1856 Collected works on scientific medicine. Meidinger, Frankfurt

Walraven C, Mamdani M, Cohn A et al 2003 Risk of subsequent thromboembolism for patients with pre-eclampsia. British Medical Journal 326:791–792

Walsh M (ed) 2002 Watson's clinical nursing and related sciences, 6th edn. Bailliere Tindall, Edinburgh

Walthall H 2006 Antiplatelet therapy in the treatment and prevention of thrombus formation. British Journal of Cardiac Nursing 1(12):568–574

Willcox A 2004 Air travel. Practice Nursing 15(4):190–192

Wilmott R, Alikhan R 2002 Venous thromboprophylaxis in acutely ill patients: nursing role. British Journal of Nursing 11(19):1248–1258

Yu C K H, Teoh T G, Robinson S 2006 Obesity in pregnancy. British Journal of Obstetrics and Gynaecology 113:1117–1125

Chapter 5

Anaemias and the haemoglobinopathies

INTRODUCTION

Anaemia is the name generally applied to a range of deficiencies in the quality or quantity of red blood cells. Anaemia and haemoglobinopathies, which are becoming more prevalent in the UK, are significant problems in pregnancy, which can have a detrimental effect on both maternal and fetal health. Midwives have an increasingly important role in the management of these conditions. It is essential, therefore, that midwives have knowledge and understanding of the pathophysiology, distinguishing clinical features and current management in order to provide a high standard of midwifery care to women and their families affected by these conditions.

RELEVANT ANATOMY AND PHYSIOLOGY

The blood

The blood is the transport system of the body, as it carries materials via blood vessels. It is a red viscous fluid consisting of two components, a fluid portion or plasma, which makes up 55–60% of blood volume, and a cellular component comprising red blood cells, white blood cells and platelets.

An average man has, circulating in his body, approximately 5.6 L of blood, 1 L in lungs, 3 L in systemic venous circulation and 1 L in heart and arteriolar circulation. A woman has approximately 4.5 L of blood and a newborn baby, conversely,

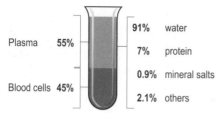

Figure 5.1   Components of blood.

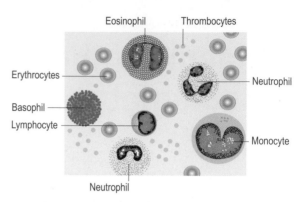

Figure 5.2   Blood cells found in plasma.

has only 250–300 mL. Blood volume can be calculated for either a man or woman by calculating 7% of body weight in kilograms (Martini 2005).

Plasma

Plasma (Fig. 5.1) is the straw coloured fluid which remains after the blood cells have been removed. It is composed of 90–95% water and plasma proteins, which are formed in the liver and have many uses: nutrients, electrolytes, hormones, enzymes and waste products.

Plasma and interstitial fluid encompass most of the volume of extracellular fluid in the body. As water, ions and small solutes are continually exchanged between interstitial fluid, capillary walls and plasma their composition is very similar (Martini 2005). The characteristic straw colour of plasma is formed from bilirubin – the main bile pigment derived from haemoglobin breakdown (Stables & Rankin 2005). Plasma contains dissolved proteins, which because of their large size and shape, cannot cross capillary walls. The main plasma proteins are albumin, globulins and fibrinogen.

Albumin accounts for approximately 60% of plasma proteins and is a contributor to osmotic pressure of plasma. It also assists in the transport of lipids and steroid hormones.

Globulins include antibodies which attack foreign proteins and pathogens, and transport globulins which are used in the transport of ions, hormones and lipids. They constitute approximately 35% of proteins in plasma.

Fibrinogen accounts for approximately 4% of plasma proteins and is essential in the clotting of blood and can be converted into insoluble fibrin. The remaining 1% is composed of specialized plasma proteins whose roles vary widely (Martini 2005).

The remaining 40–45% of blood volume is made up of the cells, most of which are erythrocytes (red blood cells) the smaller proportion remaining containing leucocytes (white blood cells) and thrombocytes (platelets). Each will be discussed in turn.

Erythrocytes

Erythrocytes (Fig. 5.2) or red blood cells are non-nucleated bi-concave discs. This unusual shape has an important effect on the function of erythrocytes. Large surface area to volume allows rapid exchange of oxygen from the cell to tissues. When passing through narrow blood vessels erythrocytes can form stacks one behind each other to smooth the flow without restriction. Additionally they are able to bend and flex when entering and squeezing through small arterioles and capillaries.

Erythrocytes are produced in the red bone marrow of the ribs, sternum, vertebrae, skull and long bones. There are approximately 4.5–5.5 million/ml^3 of blood, and they have a life span of 120 days. At the end of this time, the erythrocyte is destroyed in the spleen, liver and bone marrow.

Erythropoiesis or red cell production is stimulated by the hormone erythropoietin, mainly produced in the kidney. Erythrocytes develop from myeloid stem cells as erythroblasts, which are nucleated, and as they mature, they become reticulocytes, amass haemoglobin and lose the nucleus.

Oxygen is carried in erythrocytes bound to the protein haemoglobin (Fig. 5.3). A haemoglobin molecule consists of four polypeptide chains, with a 'haem' portion at the centre of each chain.

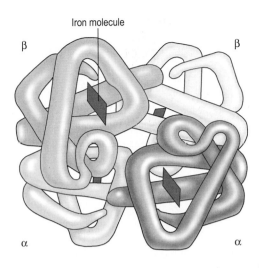

Figure 5.3   Haemoglobin molecule.

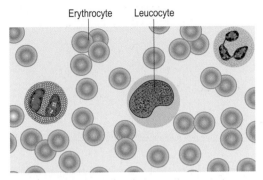

Figure 5.4   Leucocytes.

the release of erythropoietin is increased; this in turn stimulates the bone marrow to produce more erythroblasts. If the demand is excessive, immature cells such as reticulates may be released prematurely into the circulation (Hand 2001).

Estimation of the amount of haemoglobin in the circulation is a measurement of the blood's oxygen-carrying capacity. Normal levels for Hb are 11–13 g/dL for women, and 14–17 g/dL for men.

Leucocytes

Leucocytes (Fig. 5.4) (white blood cells) are nucleated cells, are much larger than red blood cells and are involved in protecting the body against disease. Leucocytes comprise 1% of the circulating blood volume. They have the ability of leaving the blood vessels to invade diseased tissues. Leucocytes are classified according to whether they are *granular* or *agranular*.

Granular leucocytes are large cells containing a nucleus and granular cytoplasm. There are three kinds: neutrophils, eosinophils and basophils. Neutrophils are highly mobile and specialize in attacking and ingesting bacteria. They have a very short life span of approximately 10 h. Eosinophils attack objects that are coated with antibodies. Through phagocytosis, they engulf antibody marked bacteria, protozoa, or cellular debris. Basophils are the rarest of the white cells and they migrate to sites of injury, where they release histamine, which acts as a vasodilator and attracts other white cells to the injury site.

Agranular leucocytes, monocytes and lymphocytes, have round or kidney-shaped nuclei and cytoplasm that lacks any granules. Monocytes become tissue macrophages. There are three

---

Box 5.1 Oxygen saturation

Each haemoglobin molecule can bind with four molecules of oxygen. Oxygen saturation is an indication of the percentage of haemoglobin saturated with oxygen. If all haemoglobin molecules contain four molecules of oxygen, oxygen saturation will be 100%. Values <90% indicate that body tissues are hypoxic. Oxygen saturation of haemoglobin molecules can be affected by an adverse internal environment, such as acidosis; this may occur when an individual has breathing difficulties, or toxins circulating in the blood stream due to acute infection. Oxygen saturation can be measured by pulse oximetry.

Each 'haem' portion is a deep red pigment that contains one iron atom bound to one oxygen molecule. Haemoglobin molecules can bind up to four oxygen molecules (Box 5.1).

Haemoglobin picks up oxygen in the lungs becoming oxyhaemoglobin and thus carries oxygen to the tissues. The cell membrane of the erythrocyte is thin and pliable and allows gaseous exchange between the cell and tissues. Haemoglobin exchanges oxygen for carbon dioxide and becomes carboxyhaemoglobin. The deoxygenated blood returns to the lungs for removal of the waste products.

If the body detects low levels of oxygen, for example at high altitude, or through anaemia,

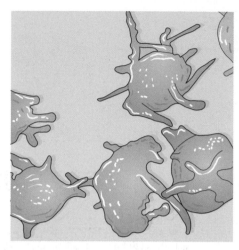

Figure 5.5 Platelets.

Table 5.1 Functions of blood

- Transports oxygen, nutrients, hormones, enzymes and chemicals to all cells
- Removes carbon dioxide and other waste products from cells
- Facilitates homeostasis by regulating body temperature
- Regulating water, electrolyte and acid base balance
- Defence against toxins and pathogens.

From Martini 2005.

different types of lymphocytes. T cells are involved in cell-mediated immunity whereas B cells are primarily responsible for humoral immunity (relating to antibodies). Some T lymphocytes act as natural killer cells and are responsible for the detection and destruction of abnormal tissue cells, for example viruses and cancers.

Leucocytes develop from stem cells in the bone marrow and mature through several stages. Lymphocytes mature in bone marrow or the thymus gland. They have varying life spans from 100 days to several years.

Thrombocytes

Thrombocytes (Fig. 5.5) (platelets) are small, sticky, granular blood cell fragments that play an essential role in the arrest of bleeding or haemostasis. They are the first line of defence against damage to blood vessels; they adhere to any defects and assist in formation of a platelet plug and a fibrin clot during the clotting process. Platelets live for 9–12 days before being destroyed by phagocytes, mainly in the spleen. There are on average 350 000 platelets/μL of circulating blood.

The blood thus contains a number of cells which give it a vital role in the normal functioning of the body (Table 5.1).

Classification of blood

The differences in human blood are due to the presence or absence of certain protein molecules called antigens and antibodies. The antigens are located on the surface of the red blood cells while the antibodies are found in the blood plasma.

ABO blood groups

There are four main blood types A, B, AB, O (Table 5.2).

1. Blood Group A: The individual, who belongs to this blood group, will have A antigens on the surface of the red blood cells and anti-B antibodies in plasma. Therefore this person can only receive blood from group A preferably, or O, but can donate blood to group A or AB.
2. Blood Group B: has B antigens on the surface of the red blood cells and anti-A antibodies in the plasma. This individual can only receive blood from group B or O and can donate blood to groups B or AB.
3. Blood Group AB: has both A and B antigens on the red blood cell and no anti-A or anti-B antibodies in the plasma. This person can receive blood from any group (universal recipient) but can only donate to group AB.
4. Blood Group O: has neither A or B antigens on the surface of the red blood cells but has both A and B antibodies in plasma. This person can only receive blood from group O, but can donate blood to any blood group A, B, AB, or O (universal donor).

When red blood cells carrying one or both antigens are exposed to the corresponding antibodies, they agglutinate; that is, clump together. People usually have antibodies against those red cell antigens that they lack. If a person is transfused with blood of

Table 5.2   ABO blood groups

ABO blood type	Antigen A	Antigen B	Antibody anti–A	Antibody anti–B
A	Yes	No	No	Yes
B	No	Yes	Yes	No
O	No	No	Yes	Yes
AB	Yes	Yes	No	No

a different group than their own, it is the reaction between the donor's red cell and the recipient's serum that causes the potentially fatal side-effects.

Rhesus factor

Rhesus (Rh) antigens are transmembrane proteins exposed at the surface of red blood cells. There are a number of different Rh antigens. Red cells that are 'Rhesus positive' express the antigen designated D. About 15% of the population have no RhD antigens and thus are 'RhD (Rhesus) negative'.

Individuals either have, or do not have, the Rhesus factor (or RhD antigen) on the surface of their red blood cells. A person is either Rhesus positive (does have the Rhesus antigen) or Rhesus negative (does not have the antigen). The anti-body anti-D does not occur normally in the serum of Rhesus negative blood. If a person receives a Rhesus positive blood transfusion or if during childbirth a woman who is Rhesus negative receives red blood cells from a Rhesus positive baby, antibodies are produced, and if in a subsequent pregnancy the fetus is Rhesus positive, maternal antibodies will cause haemolysis of fetal red blood cells, which causes anaemia and jaundice or if severe, may even cause death (Box 5.2).

Identification of the ABO and Rhesus blood grouping systems are necessary during early pregnancy to ensure safe blood transfusion where necessary, and for the detection and management of Rhesus iso-immunization.

PHYSIOLOGICAL CHANGES IN THE CARDIOVASCULAR SYSTEM AND BLOOD IN PREGNANCY

These changes develop primarily to meet the increasing metabolic demands of the mother and

Box 5.2 Haemolytic disease of the newborn

This condition occurs when there is an incompatibility between the blood groups of a mother and the fetus. Commonly, this is the result of the mother being Rhesus negative while her baby is Rhesus positive. During the birth of her first Rhesus positive baby, fetal blood cells pass into the mother's bloodstream and cause her body to produce Rhesus antibodies. With subsequent pregnancies in which the fetus is Rhesus positive, these antibodies pass across the placental barrier and destroy the Rhesus positive blood cells of the fetus. This condition is now largely preventable by the administration of anti-D immunoglobulins to the mother immediately after the birth of her first baby.

fetus. Circulating blood volume increases gradually and progressively from about 6 weeks' gestation and continues until 32–34 weeks approximately. This increased blood volume is required to supply the uterus, breasts, kidneys, skin and to a lesser extent other organs, facilitating the exchange of maternal and fetal gases and nutrients. Plasma volume is increased by approximately 40% and is greater than the increase in erythrocytes, which is approximately 20%. This results in haemodilution and consequently, a decrease in haemoglobin concentration, resulting in a physiological anaemia.

Pregnancy causes a rise in cardiac output by about 40%, due to an increase in stroke volume in early pregnancy. This results in more blood being ejected with each ventricular contraction and is maintained by a slight increase in heart rate. The increase in output occurs mainly in the first and second trimesters, with a levelling out in the third trimester.

Heart size increases to cope with increased cardiac output. Upward displacement of the diaphragm by the enlarging uterus causes the heart to be displaced to the left and rotated anteriorly.

Blood pressure remains relatively unchanged in the first trimester of pregnancy due to the increase in blood volume and cardiac output. However, the diastolic pressure may fall in the second trimester and then rise progressively in the third trimester. This is thought to be due to a decreased systemic resistance associated with the local production of vasodilatory prostaglandins.

ANAEMIA

Anaemia can be defined as a deficiency in the quality or quantity of red blood cells, with the result that oxygen-carrying capacity of the blood is reduced. Every body system is affected as organ function is impaired and deteriorates due to oxygen starvation.

Anaemia is considered to be present in a pregnant woman when haemoglobin is 11 g/dL or less. In the UK, where general health and nutrition is considered to be ever improving, some areas do not consider a woman to be anaemic until her haemoglobin level is 10 g/dL or less. A word of caution, however, with the increasing numbers of asylum seekers and people immigrating to the UK with different health status and cultural practices, it is mandatory that each woman is assessed as an individual. Globally, iron deficiency anaemia is found in 20–25 % of the world's population.

During pregnancy, there is rapid cell division and a greater demand for haemoglobin synthesis. Serum ferritin levels should remain at or above 10 µg/dL to meet the demands of the enlarging uterus and fetus.

Iron requirements during pregnancy

Extra iron is required by the body during pregnancy; the total iron demands range between 580 and 1340 mg, and of that, up to 1050 mg will be lost at birth (Hillman 1996). In early pregnancy, the requirement is approximately 2.5 mg/day and this increases to around 6.6 mg/day in the third trimester. A normal diet contains 15–20 mg of iron/day

in developed countries, and 3–10% is absorbed mainly from the duodenum. In a healthy woman, the loss of iron daily is 1–2 mg (Jordan & McOwat 2002).

Anaemia

There are two classifications of anaemia in common use, and these are often combined in clinical practice.

1. Based on cause:
   - Blood loss, which may be acute or chronic (haemorrhagic)
   - Inadequate production of normal blood cells by the bone marrow (hypoproliferic, hypoplastic, aplastic) or lacking essential factors for cell maturation
   - Excessive destruction of red blood cells (haemolytic)
   - Abnormal haemoglobin structure, which includes sickle cell disease and thalassaemia (haemoglobinopathies).
2. Based on the size of the red cells – the mean cell volume (MCV):

This second classification is very practical, as the majority of peripheral blood counts measured in the UK are analysed on contemporary electronic cell counters.

- Macrocytic (large red cells)
- Normocytic (normal sized red cells)
- Microcytic (small red cells).

Signs and symptoms of anaemia

Each type of anaemia has variable features, depending on the speed of onset but there are some common sign and symptoms, and some, but not all, will present in most cases. Women may not realize they have these symptoms until questioned, and often put their feelings of tiredness and lethargy down to the effect of pregnancy, the time of the year, or tiredness due to pressure of work and family.

Symptoms Lassitude, fatigue, irritability and breathlessness on exertion are the most common symptoms. Angular stomatitis may also occur in which painful cracks at the angle of the mouth develop, leading to loss of appetite.

Signs Pallor of skin and mucous membranes may be observed, and may be seen in the palms of hands and conjunctivae, although these are subjective and unreliable signs. In severe anaemia, presenting clinical features are directly related to insufficient oxygen supply and include tachycardia and palpitations, angina and intermittent claudication.

Anaemia in pregnancy

Iron deficiency anaemia

Iron deficiency anaemia occurs in 23% of pregnant women in developed countries and in 52% of women in developing countries (WHO et al 2001).

Predisposing factors

Poor nutrition or absorption of nutrients The aim of a good diet in pregnancy is to optimize the health of the woman and to enhance the health of the developing fetus. Malnutrition is associated with low birthweight and disease in later life. Poverty and malnutrition go hand in hand, particularly in developing countries. The best possible environment for pregnancy is where the woman is healthy with a wide varied diet and adequate nutritional stores, which will optimize maternal and fetal health.

The Western diet with refined foods can be deficient in B vitamins, especially folic acid. A vegetarian diet may need to be supplemented with iron, vitamins B and D. Conversely, some micronutrients are hazardous if overused in pregnancy, for example, vitamin A, found in liver, which is associated with birth defects, such as cleft palate and heart defects (IVAC 2006).

Maternal nutrition even in developed countries can be less than optimum, particularly where women with low income, as a result of poor education, minimum wage employment or unemployment, are unable to provide themselves with an adequate diet. It is also well known that there are many misconceptions of what constitutes a healthy diet and health education advice may be misunderstood (Blincoe 2006).

The National Institute for Clinical Excellence (NICE) published, through their Screening committee, a policy position stating that all pregnant women should be offered a test for anaemia.

This should be considered a fundamental part of antenatal care. NICE plans to publish a routine antenatal care guideline in late 2007 (National Screening Policy Position 2006).

A varied diet should contain all the food groups, with sufficient calories to maintain metabolic needs and to enable normal activity and exercise. This diet should not lead to excessive storage of fat. It should contain all the micronutrients, such as vitamins and minerals, necessary to maintain a healthy lifestyle. Foods of a low nutritional value, such as alcohol, salt and processed foods should be taken only in moderation.

Women on low incomes may not take in enough calories to meet the energy demands of pregnancy, and consequently, the intake of micronutrients may also be insufficient (Jordan & McOwat 2002). Poor nutrition can lead to the woman being less able to cope with the rigours of labour. This in turn may lead to low birthweight infants with a poor ability to cope with illness or disease.

Midwives are well placed to provide women with accurate up-to-date information on nutrition that takes into account their individual situation. It is pointless advising costly items of food where income prohibits the purchase of these items. Many other factors affect dietary habits, for example availability of particular foods, the ease or difficulty in obtaining them, eating habits, such as whether families eat as a unit, or separately, their likes and dislikes and the support of the family unit when implementing change.

Certain chronic infections and diseases cause several changes in erythropoiesis. These include a slightly shortened red blood cell life span; decreases in the amount of iron that is available in the plasma; and decreases in the activity of the bone marrow. In the presence of these three effects, a low to moderate grade anaemia may develop. The symptoms of the anaemia often go unnoticed in the face of the primary disease. Conditions associated with the anaemia of infection and chronic diseases include malaria, Crohn's disease and ulcerative colitis. A person suffering from chronic renal disease rarely achieves a pregnancy but should it occur, the disease may produce a similar anaemia because it causes reduced levels of erythropoietin – the hormone that stimulates the production of red blood cells in the bone marrow.

Treatment of the underlying disease can prevent or reverse the anaemia. Chronic diseases such as Crohn's disease are difficult to treat and patients may exhibit intermittent anaemia that varies with their condition.

Box 5.3 Hookworm

Infestation with hookworm can provoke iron deficiency and iron deficiency anaemia (Fig. 5.6). The hookworm is a parasitic worm. It thrives in warm climates, including African and American countries. The hookworm enters the body through the skin, through the soles of bare feet, where it then migrates to the small intestines and attaches itself to the villi. The hookworm damages the villi, resulting in blood loss, and they produce anticoagulants that promote continued bleeding. Each worm can provoke the loss of up to 0.25 mL of blood/day. Because of international travel and the migrant population, hookworm is increasingly likely to be seen in the UK.

Excessive or prolonged blood loss Frequent or prolonged menses or bleeding haemorrhoids can leave a woman with a less than optimal haemoglobin level and inadequate nutrient stores prior to pregnancy. If these are combined with repeated or multiple pregnancies, anaemia may quickly develop. Even a relatively minor antepartum haemorrhage may have a very serious effect on the woman's well-being.

Chronic infections such as pyelonephritis, malaria, or intestinal parasites may also lead to anaemia (Box 5.3 and Fig. 5.6). Malaria is not endemic in the UK, but approximately 2000 cases occur every year in travellers returning from malaria-endemic countries. Pregnant women should be advised against travel into such areas (Health Protection Agency 2007).

Malabsorption Malabsorption of iron may occur due to the use of alkalis to relieve heartburn. A prolonged lack of intake of vitamin C will prevent efficient absorption of dietary iron, or severe vomiting and/or diarrhoea may prevent adequate

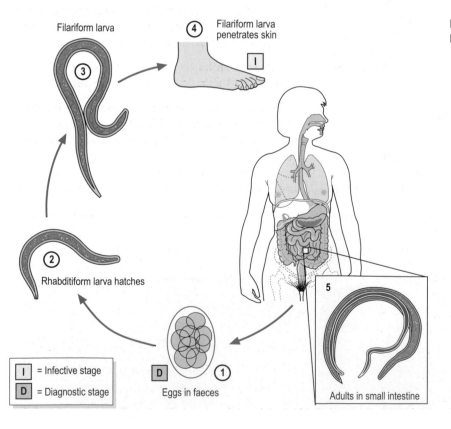

Figure 5.6 Life cycle of a hookworm.

absorption. Reduced absorption from the intestine of iron can be caused by diseases of the small intestine, such as gluten intolerance (coeliac sprue) or Crohn's disease, colorectal cancer, gastric or duodenal ulcers or aspirin; the blood loss from the digestive tract may be so slight as to be undetected on its own.

Signs and symptoms Tiredness, dizziness, fainting and pallor of mucous membranes are the most common features. In extreme cases, the nails can become brittle and spoon-shaped, with vertical stripes and a tendency to split. Sometimes a 'pica' can arise – an insatiable craving for a specific food. In other cases, brittle hair may be observed or a smooth shiny and reddened tongue, known as glossitis, may develop.

Diagnosis It is important to obtain a detailed history including appetite, diet, blood loss, or possible infection. Vegetarians may be predisposed to iron deficiency, as one of the main sources of iron is red meat. A mid-stream specimen of urine should be obtained to exclude urinary tract infection. Recurrent infections can cause anaemia. A specimen of stool should be sent to the laboratory to detect faecal occult blood which may be present if there is chronic disease of the gastrointestinal tract. A full blood count is critical to aid diagnosis (Table 5.3).

Effect of iron deficiency anaemia on pregnancy

Maternal mortality, prenatal and perinatal infant loss and prematurity are increased in untreated iron deficiency anaemia. Globally, 40% of all maternal deaths are linked to anaemia (WHO 2001). Less favourable pregnancy outcomes occur in 35–45% of women with anaemia, and their infants have less than one half of the normal iron reserves. These infants require, at an earlier age, more iron than is supplied in breast milk than their healthy counterparts. The World Health Organization also considers that up to 30% of women in the developed countries suffer from iron deficiency anaemia and this affects their earning ability, effectively trapping them in the cycle of poverty (WHO 2001).

Anaemia undermines general health and lowers the body's ability to cope with infection, and minor disorders of pregnancy may be exacerbated. Antepartum and/or postpartum haemorrhage may be rendered more serious, although it is questionable whether having iron deficiency anaemia actually increases the risk of haemorrhage. It is more likely that the woman would take longer to recover if a haemorrhage occurred.

Management during pregnancy and birth Iron therapy is usually prescribed by the GP when the blood specimen results are available. In pregnancy, where there are no contraindications, oral iron may be given, for example:

- Ferrous sulphate – 200 mg twice daily
- Ferrous gluconate – 600 mg twice daily.

All iron preparations have side-effects, for example heartburn, nausea, vomiting or constipation (BNF 2006). Women find these side-effects distressing and often stop taking iron preparations and must be given adequate information to make an informed choice. Nausea and vomiting can be

Table 5.3 Blood investigations

Haemoglobin	$\leqslant 11\,g/dL$
Packed cell volume (PCV) is the volume of red cells expressed as a fraction of the total volume of blood	Normally 35–40% in pregnancy
Mean corpuscular volume (MCV) is the average volume of a single red cell in μm^3	Normally $90\,\mu m^3$
Serum iron	60–$120\,\mu g/100\,mL$ (lowered indicates depleted iron stores)
Total iron binding capacity	325–$400\,\mu g/100\,mL$ (higher indicates depleted iron stores)
Serum ferritin	$\leqslant 10\,\mu g/dL$ (indicates exhausted iron stores)

minimized by taking the tablet with, or immediately after, food. If compliance is problematic, the midwife should advise the woman to take the medication at least 6–8h apart. Discussion with the physician may be necessary to arrange an appropriate reduction of the dosage.

The woman should be encouraged to take plenty of fruit, vegetables and water in her diet to reduce the likelihood of constipation and encourage iron absorption. Additionally, ascorbic acid (vitamin C) as a supplement (250–500mg twice daily with the iron preparation) may enhance the iron absorption.

Jordan (2002) considers that iron preparations are absorbed more effectively by the presence of acid in the stomach, and recommends that pregnant women should take their iron preparations with meat, veal or fish to stimulate gastric acid production. The midwife should also advise the woman that her stools will appear black for the duration of treatment.

Some women may require iron administered by injection when oral iron produces gastrointestinal intolerance; where there is failure of patients to cooperate in oral iron therapy; or in late pregnancy when an assured response to iron is needed as an alternative to a blood transfusion. Due to the high risks of hypersensitivity responses with these products, a test dose should be given before full administration (Ostrow & McCoy 1998). Examples of these medications include:

- Jectofer (iron sorbital citrate complex) i.m. 1.5mg/kg of body weight (100mg in 2mL ampoules)

- Imferon i.v. calculated on body weight. A test dose of 10 drops/min for 30min should be given. Infusion should then be stopped for 1h. If there is no reaction after 1h the infusion can be continued. Close observations of the patient must be carried out to detect an anaphylactic reaction. Infusion rate can be increased if there is no reaction.

In labour, blood is cross-matched in the presence of anaemia or other risk factors. Blood transfusion is the quickest method of replacing blood loss, but it is only given if there is no alternative. Plasma expanders may be used and there are two forms, crystalloid and colloid. Crystalloids include basic intravenous infusions such as normal saline, 5% glucose solution and various combinations thereof. Colloids include albumin, dextrans, starches and gelatins.

It is important to take into account religious beliefs regarding blood transfusion and particularly to ensure if a woman is a Jehovah's witness. The multidisciplinary team must be alerted of this situation preferably early in pregnancy so that alternative treatments can be fully discussed. The patient's wishes regarding blood transfusion can then be recorded in her medical and midwifery notes along with other possible courses of action if required (NMC 2005).

Midwives' role Midwives need to be alert for the signs of anaemia and be able to initiate appropriate action, including interpreting blood specimen results, critically evaluating available evidence and notifying medical colleagues as and where necessary.

The midwife should support, inform and educate women on care in pregnancy. She should have knowledge and understanding of the clinical features of anaemia, and current management, including available drug therapy. Liaison with the GP is paramount, in order to provide effective up-to-date care, and should include other members of the multidisciplinary team as appropriate.

Communication skills are, as always, paramount. Dietary advice must be appropriate for social, religious and cultural backgrounds; it should be practical and provided at a level that the woman can understand. Poor dietary habits and food fads are common, and support and positive encouragement must be given to effect change, however small. Criticism and censure is counterproductive and will only succeed in alienating the woman and achieve nothing. Maternal nutrition has been seen as an undervalued factor in pregnancy care, but in the treatment of iron deficiency anaemia, a balanced varied diet can reduce perinatal loss and prematurity as well as maternal morbidity. All observations and advice should be recorded within midwifery notes (NMC 2005).

Folic acid deficiency anaemia

Folic acid, a 'B' group vitamin, is necessary for the formation of nuclei in all body cells. In pregnancy, the demands of the fetus and placental growth may cause a deficiency of folic acid, unless the intake is increased.

Deficiency of folic acid causes a megaloblastic anaemia, where large, irregular shaped, immature, nucleated, red blood cells called megaloblasts, circulate in the blood. Megaloblasts are normally only present in bone marrow. A concurrent deficiency in leucocytes and thrombocytes may also be determined.

Women most at risk of folic acid deficiency include malnourished women, multiparous women, or women with a multiple pregnancy. Women having drug therapies, or certain anticonvulsants (such as phenytoin and phenobarbital) and drugs used to treat ulcerative colitis such as sulfasalazine also decrease the absorption of this vitamin. Trimethoprim-sulfamethoxazole (an antibiotic) also interferes with the metabolism of folic acid.

Alcohol consumed in large amounts interferes with the absorption and processing (metabolism) of folic acid and this should be considered when caring for a pregnant woman with alcohol abuse. Neural tube defects have been clearly demonstrated to have a link with low folic acid intake (DOH 1992). All pregnant women and those intending to become pregnant are advised to take 0.4–4mg folic acid daily. Foods containing folic acid are green leafy vegetables, for example, broccoli or spinach.

Clinical features   The general features of anaemia may be present, including fatigue, shortness of breath, dizziness, and glossitis. If blood specimens indicate macrosomic anaemia, then the folic acid levels should be estimated.

Management of folic acid deficiency anaemia For management of folic acid deficiency anaemia, 5–10mg folic acid orally daily may be prescribed. If there is severe folic acid anaemia, the drug may be administered intravenously.

Midwives' role   A clear accurate history must be obtained including dietary and lifestyle habits. Information and explanation should be provided regarding the importance of folic acid in early pregnancy. Where alcohol misuse is identified, the physician may prescribe larger doses of folic acid. Some studies have indicated that administration

of folic acid and antiepileptic drugs such as carbamazepine, phenytoin, barbiturates and primidone have resulted in increased seizure frequency (Guidolin et al 1998). Midwives should advise women with epilepsy to consult their medical practitioners prior to commencing folic acid to adjust antiepileptic drug dosages.

Vitamin B_{12} (hydroxocobalamin) deficiency

Vitamin B_{12} is a member of the vitamin B complex. This is a water soluble vitamin which cannot be stored for long in the body. It contains cobalt, and is also known as cobalamin. It is exclusively synthesized by bacteria and is found primarily in meat, eggs and dairy products. In order for vitamin B_{12} to be absorbed by the body, it must bind to the intrinsic factor, secreted by cells in the stomach. When given in oral doses ranging from 0.1–2mg daily, vitamin B_{12} can be absorbed in a pathway that does not require an intact ileum or intrinsic factor (Oh & Brown 2003).

Vitamin B_{12} is essential for blood cell production and normal nervous system functioning. Vitamin B_{12}'s primary function is in the formation of erythrocytes, and it is necessary (along with folic acid) for the rapid synthesis of DNA during cell division. This is especially important in tissues where cells are dividing rapidly, particularly the bone marrow tissues responsible for red blood cell formation. If deficiency occurs, DNA production is disrupted and a megaloblastic anaemia results.

Deficiency is rare in pregnancy, but lactating women should ensure a good supply of vitamin B_{12}. Causes of vitamin B_{12} deficiency include a diet low in vitamin B_{12}, for example, a strict vegetarian diet that excludes all meat, fish, dairy products and eggs. Chronic alcoholism, abdominal or intestinal surgery that affects intrinsic factor production or absorption, may lead to this deficiency, as does Crohn's disease, intestinal malabsorption disorders and fish tapeworm.

Management   Vitamin B_{12} replacement therapy is given as hydroxocobalamin 100µg i.m. every second day for 6 doses, then every 3 months if pernicious anaemia is diagnosed. If deficiency is due to dietary deficiency, treatment is given initially by intramuscular injection until normal levels are reached then replaced by oral therapy.

Several studies have indicated that oral cobalamin is as effective as the parenteral form including Graham et al (2007) and Nyholm et al (2003), who concluded that many physicians were unaware of previous research and trials and that oral therapy is an underutilized treatment for B_{12} deficiency.

Midwives' role Midwives should be able to advise women in the sources of vitamin B_{12} – free-range eggs or half a pint of milk (full fat or semi-skimmed) contains $1.2\,\mu g$ of this vitamin. A slice of vegetarian cheddar cheese $(40\,g)$ contains $0.5\,\mu g$. A boiled egg contains $0.7\,\mu g$. Fermentation in the manufacture of yoghurt destroys much of the B_{12} present. Boiling milk can also destroy much of the B_{12}.

Vegans are recommended to ensure their diet includes foods fortified with vitamin B_{12}. A range of B_{12} fortified foods are available. These include yeast extracts, vegetable stock, 'veggie-burger' mixes, textured vegetable protein, soya milks, vegetable and sunflower margarines and breakfast cereals.

The midwife should keep in close contact with the woman to ensure therapy is effective, and advise the woman to ensure good dietary intake. It must be explained that the full effect of the drug therapy is a gradual process, and not instantaneous. The midwife should liaise with the medical practitioner where non-compliance or other problems emerge. All care should be recorded in appropriate documents (NMC 2005).

G6PD deficiency

G6PD deficiency is caused by a defect in the production of glucose-6-phosphate dehydrogenase (an enzyme present in red blood cells) in the blood, which can cause a haemolytic anaemia. Globally, it affects over 400 million people and is the most common human enzyme defect (Hamilton et al 2004).

G6PD deficiency is a recessive sex-linked trait. Thus, males have only one copy of the G6PD gene, but females have two copies. Recessive genes are masked in the presence of a gene that encodes normal G6PD. Accordingly, females with one copy of the gene for G6PD deficiency are usually normal, while males with one copy have the trait.

Males who inherit an abnormal gene are invariably affected. Heterozygote females usually have approximately 50% G6PD enzyme activity. The degree of the G6PD deficiency depends on the amount of the enzyme which is missing. The disorder occurs most frequently in individuals of Mediterranean, African and Asian origin.

G6PD deficiency reduces energy available to maintain the integrity of the red cell membrane, which shortens erythrocyte survival. Presentation is usually with an acute episode of intravascular haemolysis on exposure to certain drugs, infection or acute illness. The condition is also known as favism as sudden haemolysis may be precipitated by the ingestion of (broad) fava beans.

Women should receive genetic counselling in the antenatal period; pregnancy, labour and delivery are usually normal. Neonates born with G6PD deficiency are more likely to develop prolonged jaundice (Stables & Rankin 2005) and prenatal screening should be carried out to prevent future haemolytic episodes.

Haemoglobinopathies

Haemoglobinopathies are inherited conditions in which the normal adult haemoglobin (HbA) is wholly, or partially, replaced by one or more abnormal types.

The main haemoglobinopathies, fall into three groups:

1. Sickle cell disease: Abnormalities of the protein (globin) structure, resulting in synthesis of abnormal haemoglobin (Hoffbrand et al 2002).
2. Thalassaemia: Imbalanced globin chain production, due to a reduced or absent rate of synthesis (Bennet 1996, Proven et al 1997 cited in Khattab et al 2006).
3. HbS/β-thalassaemia: A combination of sickle cell and thalassaemia, where there is an abnormality of the globin structure combined with a reduced rate of synthesis.

These conditions are most common among people whose ancestral origin can be traced to malarial areas of the world, although population movement and relationships between members of different groups has resulted in changed patterns of occurrence.

Within the UK, England has the most multi-racial society, and sickle cell trait and thalassaemia are among England's most commonly inherited genetic disorders. Sickle cell trait affects an estimated 170 000 people in the UK (Allen 2005), with an estimated 240 000 carriers. Around 700 people are affected by major thalassaemia, with an estimated 214 000 carriers (NHS Sickle Cell & Thalassaemia Screening Programme 2004).

Sickle cell disease

The Sickle Cell Society (2005) state that 'Sickle cell is a condition that affects the normal oxygen carrying capacity of red blood cells. The symptoms can include severe anaemia, intense pain, damage to major organs and infections. These episodic periods of pain are sometimes called 'crises'. Although there is no routine cure for sickle cell, it can be managed to reduce the frequency and severity of crises and their complications by prompt recognition and treatment'.

There are over 300 different types of haemoglobin (Sickle Cell Society 2005) and the most common type is haemoglobin (Hb)A, which consists of a protein, globin and two alpha and two beta polypeptide chains. Haemoglobin A is inherited as the homozygous (pair of genes which are the same) form from both parents – Mother HbA, Father HbA = Child HbAA.

Sickle cell disease is the family of haemoglobin disorders in which both Hb beta chains are abnormal, with one or both of the Hb beta chain genes having the sickle mutation (HbS). Sickle cell anaemia occurs when HbS is inherited from both parents. Mother HbS, Father HbS = Child HbSS (European Haemoglobinopathy Registry 2003, Weatherall 1997).

PEGASUS (Professional Education for Genetic Assessment and Screening) is a useful resource for health professionals to develop their knowledge in basic genetics through education and training with interactive online learning and courses for those involved in antenatal and newborn screening (PEGASUS 2007). PEGASUS is a national collaboration led by the University of Nottingham Division Of Primary Care and funded by the NHS Sickle Cell and Thalassaemia Screening Programme acting on behalf of the National Screening Committee.

The incidence of these disorders is thought to be increasing perhaps mainly due to increased uptake from screening campaigns and prolonged life span of sufferers through more effective treatments. Prevalence of the disorder is not restricted to the black African-Caribbean population (1–10), but also includes West Africans and Asians (1–50 sufferers), Greeks, Italians and those of other Mediterranean origins (1–100 sufferers) (De 2005). Increasing inter-racial marriage or partnership emphasizes that in the future, screening for these conditions cannot be restricted to ethnic minorities alone. There is a dearth of educational material and training resources available, particularly outwith England (Khattab et al 2006).

Sickle cell trait

If one of the sickle cell genes carries the instructions to make sickle haemoglobin (HbS) and the other carries the instructions to make normal haemoglobin (HbA) then the person has sickle cell trait and is a carrier of the sickle haemoglobin gene. People with the sickle cell trait do not have any of the clinical features associated with sickle cell anaemia. They are usually healthy, but according to the Sickle Cell Society may require extra oxygen during anaesthesia and surgical operations. They are also advised against participating in strenuous sports where oxygen supply may be reduced. If both parents are carriers, there is a 1 in 4 chance that each of their children could be born with sickle cell anaemia. Sickle cell trait offers some protection against malaria (Box 5.4).

Sickle cell disease

Sickle cell disease is present from birth but signs and symptoms are rare before 3–6 months of age. Normal red blood cells can bend and flex quite easily when they pass through arteries, arterioles and capillaries, but sickled cells are rigid and unable to bend or flex in the same manner. Haemoglobin molecules normally exist as disc-shaped isolated units in the red blood cell, whether they are transporting oxygen or not.

Sickle haemoglobin molecules also exist as isolated units in the red blood cells when they are transporting O_2, but when the cells release the O_2 to the tissues, the molecules tend to stick

Box 5.4 Protection from malaria

People with normal haemoglobin are susceptible to death from malaria. People with sickle cell disease are susceptible to death from the complications of sickle cell disease. People with sickle cell trait, who have one gene for haemoglobin A and one gene for haemoglobin S, have a greater chance of surviving malaria and do not suffer adverse consequences from the haemoglobin S gene.

The *Plasmodium falciparum* parasite causes a severe form of malaria, but in those with both normal and abnormal haemoglobin, sickle cell trait, when the parasite enters the abnormal Hb cells they quickly sickle; the cells are then destroyed by phagocytosis and removed from the circulation by the spleen (Pallister 1992). Thus, the individual is less seriously affected by malaria.

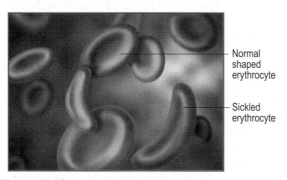

Figure 5.7   Sickled erythrocytes.

together and form long chains or polymers. These polymers or rods distort the cell and cause it to bend out of shape and it becomes sickle or crescent shaped (Fig. 5.7) – hence the name (British Committee for Standards in Haematology 2003). On returning to the lungs, the cells become oxygenated, and they then regain their normal disc shape. This cyclic alteration in the shape of the molecules damages the haemoglobin and eventually the erythrocyte itself. The cells become rigid and fail to move through the microcirculation, blocking blood flow to a microscopic region of tissue. Amplified many times, these episodes produce tissue hypoxia, resulting in pain and tissue damage or necrosis (De 2005).

The increased mechanical fragility and surface abnormalities of the cells containing sickle haemoglobin reduce the red cell life span from the normal 120 days down to 10–30 days. The erythrocytes become easily damaged and destroyed. To combat this, the production of red cells by the bone marrow increases dramatically but is unable to keep pace with the destruction of the red cells and anaemia results.

In addition, a low blood pH occurs due to decreased clearance of carbon dioxide by the lungs. Haemoglobin levels vary between 7–10 g/dL and the blood picture shows cells of varying maturity and size with a raised reticulocyte count due to haemolysis. Reticulocytes are young, just mature red blood cells, released by the bone marrow in response to an anaemic state, that normally comprise about 1% of the red cells in the human body.

Clinical features   The clinical features of sickle cell anaemia result from increased blood viscosity and vascular obstruction by deformed, sickled red cells. The main symptoms are anaemia, pain or infection. Disruption of blood flow causes vascular occlusions, haemorrhages and ischaemic necrosis in tissues and organs throughout the body. Pain episodes are believed to be caused by an inflammatory response to ischaemia, necrosis and the stasis of the flow of blood in the micro-circulation. Problems associated with pain include haematuria, kidney damage, and orthopaedic problems involving bone.

Diagnosis   Sickle cell disease may be diagnosed in childhood, or through family history. For a complete and accurate diagnosis, the definitive test used to diagnose sickle cell syndromes is haemoglobin electrophoresis. Women who have the condition or who are sickle cell carriers, and who attend for antenatal care may be fully aware of the issues and potential outcomes. Other women may have no knowledge of the condition or its implications. All women will require counselling and support.

Management of sickle cell disease   Comprehensive management of this condition involves a multidisciplinary team, including specialist doctors, nurses and medical social workers. A screening programme was introduced in England in 2004 called the NHS Sickle Cell & Thalassaemia Screening Programme enabling infants diagnosed with the condition to receive medical care at an early stage and thereby improve the quality of their lives.

Many midwives have specialized in the care of women with sickle cell disease in pregnancy. Other disciplines may also become involved in emergency situations. Survival of individuals has been vastly improved by preventive measures, for example, genetic counselling, newborn screening, vaccinations and education.

A prime objective would be to ensure the patient has as normal a life as possible while taking precautions to prevent sickle cell crisis. Good nutrition and keeping warm is essential. Some studies have emphasized the importance of a high fluid intake, and the importance, where possible, of avoiding infection (Sickle Cell Society 2005). The patient's liver and kidney function is monitored. Folic acid supplements and prophylactic antibiotic therapy may be advised. The patient should avoid situations likely to precipitate a painful episode or crisis.

Hydroxycarbamide (hydroxyurea) is a chemotherapeutic agent with potent effects on bone marrow; it is known to stimulate the body to make fetal haemoglobin, a form that normally disappears from a baby's bloodstream soon after birth. The fetal haemoglobin prevents the clumping of sickle haemoglobin. Its use is not advised in pregnancy.

Conditions likely to precipitate a crisis include:

- Strenuous exercises
- Anaesthetics
- Dehydration
- Infection
- Emotional stress
- Sudden change in temperature
- Fever
- Pregnancy and/or labour.

All of the above conditions may result in a reduction of the oxygen levels in the blood, and may lead to episodes of pain or anaemia. A crisis may occur as a result of infection. Some people have frequent crises, others are more fortunate, and have attacks only every few years. Most crises occur in childhood.

Depending on the severity, some sickle cell crises may be managed at home with analgesia and increased fluid intake. If hyperpyrexia, or severe pain in chest, spine or abdomen occurs, the patient will be admitted to hospital where adequate opiate analgesia, intravenous fluids and antibiotic therapy is supplied. In very severe instances, where the onset is rapid with abdominal pain, shock and dyspnoea, the patient is admitted to an intensive care unit, where in addition to the measures outlined above oxygen therapy and blood transfusion may be required. If acute splenic sequestration occurs, where sickle cells are trapped, causing rapid fall in Hb and enlargement of the spleen, correction of hypovolaemia followed by an emergency splenectomy may be necessary (Eckman & Platt 2004).

Effect on pregnancy

Preconception care   Ideally, couples should attend for preconception care so that they can optimize health prior to conception and also identify risks related to pregnancy. Genetic counselling may be offered but is not always taken up. In many cultures, there is a strong value placed on motherhood but women may not be in a position to make active empowered choices due to gender and social issues. In one study (Asgharian et al 2003), the authors concluded that informed reproductive decision-making was both complicated and challenging and that there was no guarantee of a successful outcome.

If the husband or partner's sickle cell status is unknown, testing may be offered to predict risk to the baby. This is not an easy choice. If prenatal diagnosis indicates the fetus is affected then the couple are faced with the dilemma of having an affected infant or to choose to terminate the pregnancy (Table 5.4). Some couples choose to have IVF and implantation of a normal fetus (Xu et al 1999).

Table 5.4 Risks associated with sickle cell anaemia	
Maternal	**Fetal**
• Reduced fertility	• IUGR
• Abortion and stillbirth	• Low birthweight
• Anaemia	
• Infection	
• Crises	
• Pre-eclampsia	
• Pre-term labour	

Antenatal management   There are approximately 1 in 400 women at risk of sickle cell disease in pregnancy in the UK. Care of women in pregnancy requires a multidisciplinary approach. The woman should be seen in a specialist centre and cared for by an obstetrician and a haematologist, as well as by a midwife. Haemoglobin electrophoresis and liver function tests are carried out in addition to normal antenatal blood investigations. Chorionic villous sampling may be offered between 11 and 13 weeks to provide fetal diagnosis. Information and explanation of the risks of this procedure must be given to facilitate informed choice. Ethical religious and cultural considerations require understanding, support and counselling.

All infection must be treated aggressively. Women with sickle cell trait have an increased incidence of bacteriuria during pregnancy (Hassell 2006). Urinary tract infections (UTI) are common and a midstream specimen of urine should be obtained immediately there is any concern. If a UTI does occur, it should be treated with a broad spectrum antibiotic, analgesia, high fluid intake, and if necessary, oxygen therapy to reduce sickling.

Pre-term labour with resultant low birthweight is also problematic. Folic acid is advised throughout pregnancy to facilitate sufficient erythrocyte production. Iron preparations are not prescribed in case of iron overload. If severe anaemia occurs, blood transfusion may be advisable.

Midwifery care must be supportive, and home visits should be offered in between hospital appointments. Forming a relationship with trust takes time, and midwives should have sufficient knowledge of the condition to facilitate the woman in making an informed choice, or to discuss issues with the woman as a partner in care. Facilitating informed choice means providing information and explanation, in a professional non-judgemental manner, related to the condition in order that the woman (and her partner) can make truly autonomous decisions about care.

Furthermore, the midwife should be able to direct the woman and her family to other relevant support agencies as required. Planning for labour and delivery, even though it should take place in a specialist unit, is paramount and the woman's choices must be discussed realistically and documented. Knowledge of labour and delivery, if discussed honestly but sensitively, can allay fears and reduce stress.

Labour and birth   Labour must be in a specialist obstetric unit with haematological and anaesthetic facilities. It is important that the woman remains well hydrated throughout labour. An intravenous infusion should be commenced, and blood crossed-matched as a precautionary measure. In some units, prophylactic antibiotic therapy is provided. All urine specimens are analysed for protein, as this finding may indicate a developing crisis.

Analgesia is important, as a frightened woman becomes stressed and this may precipitate a crisis; therefore epidural anaesthesia is the preferred choice. Blood specimens are obtained 6-hourly to estimate haemoglobin and packed cell volume (PCV) levels. Oxygen is given freely to prevent sickling and to improve cardiac function. Caesarean section is only indicated for obstetric reasons, because it provides a higher risk of thromboembolism in an already at risk population (Dent 2001).

Indications for transfusion during pregnancy and labour, remembering that repeated transfusions may lead to iron overdosage, include anaemia associated with cardiac or respiratory compromise and severe sickle cell disease (SCD)-related complications, e.g. acute chest syndrome. The benefits to the pregnancy have to be weighed against the disadvantage of transfusion (Dent 2001).

Postnatal care   The midwife should be alert for any signs of a crisis, however early ambulation and the use of antiembolic stockings (TEDS) is advised to reduce the incidence of thromboembolism. Fluid intake must be encouraged to ensure good hydration. Breast-feeding should be encouraged and this will also be facilitated by good hydration.

Anaemia, if detected must be treated without delay. The use of hydroxycarbamide (hydroxyurea), which induces fetal haemoglobin production, should be considered. Contraceptive advice should be given prior to leaving hospital and at the 6-week examination. Families should be given information regarding bone marrow transplants.

The newborn infant should be provided with screening, to identify babies with the condition, so that treatment can be started before 3 months of age (NHS Sickle Cell & Thalassaemia Screening Programme 2004).

Thalassaemia

Thalassaemias are autosomal recessive inherited conditions, where the gene is located on one of the autosomes (chromosome pairs 1–22) and affect both males and females. In a recessive condition, the infant inherits a gene for the trait from each parent. These conditions occur mainly in people of African-Caribbean, Chinese, Asian and Mediterranean origin, but with mobile populations and inter-marriage, the conditions may occur increasingly in other populations. The variety of ethnic origins in Northern European countries is increasing and poses a problem for screening and accurate diagnosis (Old 2007). Interestingly, a sporadic gene incidence (approximately 1:1000) has been found in people with Irish or Scottish ancestry (Bennet 1996).

Haemoglobin is made of the protein, globin and two alpha and two beta polypeptide chains. Each chain is a globular protein subunit which contains a single molecule of 'haem', an iron containing pigment to which one molecule of oxygen can become attached. When a person inherits the normal haemoglobin A from each parent, they will have two beta genes, one each from the mother and one from the father. They will also have four alpha genes, one pair from each parent. These people have normal healthy erythrocytes and haemoglobin.

There are a number of different types of thalassaemia caused by an imbalance of either the alpha or beta chain. In thalassaemia, one of the chains is either deleted, which is usual in alpha thalassaemia, or in other types, insufficient amounts are produced, or the chain undergoes a small deletion or other mutation resulting in an abnormal structure as may be found in beta thalassaemia (Bain 2001).

Alpha thalassaemia The inheritance of one or more faulty genes from one or both parents causing a reduction of alpha globin chains results in alpha thalassaemia. The number of faulty genes inherited will determine the type and severity of the thalassaemia condition and the less alpha chains produced, the more severe the condition.

Table 5.5	Possible genotypes
Genotype	Clinical syndrome
□ –/□ □	Silent carrier or mild alpha thalassaemia minor; alpha + thalassaemia trait
□ –/□ –	Homozygous alpha + thalassaemia or – –/□ □ thalassaemia trait
□ –/– –	Haemoglobin H disease
– –/– –	Hydrops fetalis or homozygous alpha thalassaemia; Barts haemoglobin

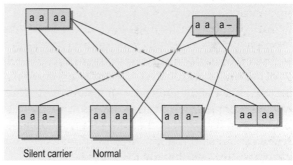

Figure 5.8 Inheritance of thalassaemia.

In the silent carrier, one parent has lost a single alpha gene. In each pregnancy, there is a (2:4) 50% chance that the fetus may inherit all four alpha genes – a normal genotype and a (2:4) 50% chance that the fetus will be a silent carrier for alpha thalassaemia (Table 5.5 and Fig. 5.8).

This type of thalassaemia is also called alpha(2) thalassaemia (Haemoglobinopathy Registry 2003). Silent carriers are healthy individuals without anaemia. Individuals who have thalassaemia trait are also healthy with perhaps mild microcytic hypochromic anaemia, but if either of these individuals plans to have a family, there is a chance that the fetus could inherit the disease state.

Haemoglobin H disease occurs when there is a deletion or inactivation of three alpha globin genes (– –/a–), and may also be termed alpha thalassaemia intermedia, with mildly to moderately severe anaemia, splenomegaly, jaundice and abnormal erythrocyte levels. When peripheral blood films are stained and examined, unusual inclusions in the erythrocytes can be seen. These inclusions represent beta chain polymers (HbH), which are unstable and precipitate in the cell, giving it the appearance of a golf ball. These inclusions are termed Heinz bodies (Yaish 2005).

Haemoglobin H disease may present differently in each individual, although blood transfusion is usually unnecessary in the majority of women (Bennet 1996, Weatherall & Clegg 2001).

Alpha thalassaemia major This condition is the result of complete deletion of a gene cluster on both copies of chromosome 16 ($- -/- -$), leading to the severe form of homozygous alpha thalassaemia, which is usually incompatible with life and results in hydrops fetalis unless intrauterine blood transfusion is given.

Beta thalassaemia Beta thalassaemia is also seen most commonly in people who originate from the Mediterranean islands, Asia, or the Middle or Far East. Again, due to inter-marriage and the mobility of populations through migration, it is seen today in many other parts of the world including the UK (Atkin & Ahmad 2000). Beta thalassaemia is similar to alpha thalassaemia in that several forms are now recognized.

Beta thalassaemia trait If a woman has a beta thalassaemia trait, she will have one chain with a correct copy of her alpha or beta chain and one copy which is faulty. She may have a mild anaemia, but mainly she will be in good health. If her partner also has the beta thalassaemia trait and they embark on a pregnancy, then there is a 1 in 4 chance of each child developing the serious disorder beta thalassaemia major. Prenatal testing and genetic counselling will be offered as necessary.

Pregnancy and thalassaemia The prevalence of thalassaemia is less common than sickle cell disease, and women with thalassaemia may or may not be fully aware that they have thalassaemia or of its severity. Care must be provided throughout the pregnancy by an obstetrician and a specialist in haematology and the haemoglobinopathies. If suspected from history, the physician will confirm the diagnosis by haemoglobin electrophoresis.

The partner or husband's status must also be ascertained in order that the correct diagnosis is reached. The genetic implications will be explained fully and prenatal diagnosis may be offered. The woman and her partner may have to make a decision whether to proceed with the pregnancy in light of the diagnosis, or to terminate. Many couples elect to continue with an affected pregnancy. Some couples undertake IVF in order to ensure implantation of a normal fetus (Xu et al 1999). This is a difficult and harrowing time and counselling will be offered by a trained midwife or other health professional.

The midwife's role is supportive and non-judgemental and she must liaise with the multidisciplinary team, so that the woman and her partner's wishes and concerns must be met. She should be able to supply information on the condition, screening and counselling centres, as well as providing information of the importance of prenatal testing and diagnosis. A relationship should be developed where trust and confidentiality are assured.

During pregnancy, some women with beta thalassaemia trait may develop an iron deficiency anaemia, which may not respond to oral therapy, and if severe, may require blood transfusion. In many women pregnancy, labour and birth proceed as normal. Newborn screening is offered to identify babies with the condition, so that treatment can be commenced before 3 months of age (NHS Sickle Cell & Thalassaemia Screening Programme 2004).

If diagnosed with beta thalassaemia major, which is the most severe form of thalassaemia the management will be as follows.

Beta thalassaemia major (Cooley's anaemia) In this instance, each gene in both chains is affected. This results in a severe debilitating illness and the infant may have a short life span, either dying in early childhood, or surviving with a life-threatening anaemia. The kidney increases erythropoietin production because of the hypoxia caused by the anaemia, stimulating red blood cell production. This leads to bone marrow expansion and increased iron absorption. The iron is deposited in the myocardium, liver and pancreas, inducing organ injury and heart failure (Hand 2001).

In the past, patients with beta thalassaemia died of heart failure. Current treatment has increased the life span quite considerably, by 10–20 years. Regular blood transfusions are the only available current management and have to be repeated frequently; approximately every month. Following the blood transfusion, the red blood cell population is again slowly broken down and destroyed. The iron content is not excreted but stays in the body. Iron overload from repeated blood transfusions can cause organ failure or death in early adult life, and chelation (iron removing) therapy must be provided to prevent this occurrence. The dose and means of delivery varies according to the needs of the patient. Oral chelating agents are being developed.

Diabetes, thyroid and adrenal disorders can also occur because of iron overload. In severe cases, exercise intolerance, bony deformities and hepatosplenomegaly may occur. Bone marrow transplantation may be considered for suitable children.

While diagnosis and management of anaemia and haemoglobinopathies are ultimately the responsibility of the obstetrician and physician, the midwife can, with careful observation and care, identify factors, in some instances, which can speed up this process, or indeed, help reduce the distress and pain, through timely intervention to the women in her care. The midwife must not undervalue her contribution, as it can be pivotal in ensuring all facets of care are provided through liaison and communication verbally and through record keeping, with all members of the multidisciplinary team.

REFERENCES

Allen S 2005 Understanding sickle cell anaemia. Pharmaceutical Journal 275:25–28

Asgharian A, Anie K, Berger M 2003 Women with sickle cell trait: reproductive decision making. Journal of Reproductive Psychology 21(1):23–34

Atkin K, Ahmad W I U 2000 Family care-giving and chronic illness: how parents cope with a child with sickle cell disorder or thalassaemia. Health Society Care in the Community 8(1):57–69

Bain B J 2001 Haemoglobinopathy diagnosis: The a, b, g, and d thalassaemias and related conditions. Blackwell, London, Ch. 3

Bennet L 1996 Thalassaemia. Supplement on haemoglobinopathies. Practice Nursing 7(1):28–30

Blincoe A J 2006 Optimum maternal nutrition for a healthy pregnancy. British Journal of Midwifery 14(3):151–154

British Committee for Standards in Haematology 2003 Guidelines for management of acute painful crisis in sickle cell disease. British Journal of Haematology 120(5):744–752

British National Formulary 2006 British National Formulary (BNF) No 50. British Medical Association and the Royal Pharmaceutical Society of Great Britain, London

De D 2005 Sickle cell anaemia 1: Background, causes and incidence in the UK. British Journal of Nursing 14(8):447–450

Dent K 2001 Perinatal review. Sickle cell disease. West Midlands Perinatal Institute, Birmingham

Department of Health 1992 Folic acid and the prevention of neural tube defects. Report from an Expert Advisory Group. Department of Health Publications Unit, Heywood

Eckman J, Platt A. 2004 Sickle Cell Information Centre – Problem Oriented Clinical Guidelines. The Sickle Cell Foundation of Georgia. University School of Medicine, Department of Paediatrics, Atlanta

European Haemoglobinopathy Register 2003 Haematology Department, Central Middlesex Hospital. The North West London Hospitals NHS Trust/Imperial College Medical School, London

Graham I D, Jette N, Tetroe J, Robinson N, Milne S, Mitchell S L 2007 Oral cobalamin remains medicine's best kept secret. Archives of Gerontology and Geriatrics 44(1):49–59

Guidolin L, Vignoli A, Canger R 1998 Worsening in seizure frequency and severity in relation to folic acid administration. In: Jordan S (ed) Pharmacology for midwives. Palgrave, Houndmills

Haemoglobinopathy Registry 2003 Haematology Department, Central Middlesex Hospital. The North West Hospitals NHS Trust. Associated University Imperial College Medical School, London

Hamilton J W, Jones F G, McMullin M F 2004 Glucose-6-phosphate dehydrogenase Guadalajara – a case of chronic non-spherocytic haemolytic anaemia responding to splenectomy and the role of splenectomy in this disorder. Hematology 9(4):307–309

Hand H 2001 Blood and the classification of anaemia: Nursing Standard 15(39):45–56

Hassell K 2006 Haemoglobinopathies in pregnancy. Current Women's Health Reviews 2(1):41–49

Health Protection Agency 2007 Malaria treatment guidelines: Malaria Reference Laboratory, London School of Hygiene and Tropical Medicine, London

Hillman R 1996 Haematopoietic agents. In: Jordan S (ed) Pharmacology for midwives. Palgrave, Houndmills

Hoffbrand M R, Petit J E, Moss P A H 2002 Essential haematology, 4th edn. Blackwell Science, Oxford

IVAC Statement 2006 Safe dose of vitamin A during pregnancy and lactation. IVAC Secretariat, International Life Sciences Institute, Research Foundation, Washington DC

Jordan S 2002 Pharmacology for midwives. Palgrave, Houndmills

Jordan S, McOwat R 2002 Nutritional supplements in pregnancy: iron and folic acid. In: Jordan S (ed) Pharmacology for midwives. Palgrave, Houndmills

Khattab A D, Rawlings B, Ali I S 2006 Care of patients with haemoglobin abnormalities: history and biology. British Journal of Nursing 15(18):994–998

Martini F H 2005 Anatomy and physiology. Pearson Education, San Francisco

National Screening Committee Policy Position 2006 All pregnant women should be offered a test for anaemia. National Collaborating Centre for Women's and Children's Health. Commissioned by the National Institute for Clinical Excellence. NICE, London

NHS Sickle Cell & Thalassaemia Screening Programme 2004 Division of Health and Social Care Research, King's College, London

NMC 2005 Guidelines for records and record keeping. Nursing and Midwifery Council, London

Nyholm P, Turpin D, Swain B et al 2003 Oral vitamin B_{12} can change your practice. Journal of Postgraduate Medicine 79:219

Oh R, Brown D 2003 Vitamin B_{12} deficiency. American Family Physician 67(5):211–237

Old J M 2007 Screening and genetic diagnosis of haemoglobinopathies. Scandinavian Journal of Clinical Laboratory Investigation 67(1):71–86

Ostrow C L, McCoy C A 1998 Hematinic agents. In: Williams B, Baer C (eds) Essentials of clinical pharmacology in nursing. Springhouse Corporation, Springhouse, Pennsylvania

Pallister C 1992 A 'crisis' that can be overcome: Management of sickle cell disease. Professional Nurse 7(8):509–513

Professional Education for Genetics Assessment and Screening 2007 University of Nottingham (on behalf of PEGASUS), Nottingham. Online. Available at: http://www.pegasus.nhs.uk (accessed April 2007)

Sickle Cell Society 2005 Sickle Cell Society, 54 Station Road, London NW10 4UA. Online. Available at: info@sicklecellsociety.org

Stables D, Rankin J 2005 Physiology in childbearing, 2nd edn. Elsevier, Edinburgh

Weatherall D J 1997 ABC of clinical haematology: the hereditary anaemias. British Medical Journal 314:492–494

Weatherall D J, Clegg J B 2001 Inherited haemoglobin disorders: an increasing global health problem. Bulletin of the World Health Organization 79(8):704–712

WHO, UNICEF, United Nations University 2001 Iron deficiency anaemia: assessment, prevention and control. World Health Organization, Geneva

Xu K, Shi Z M, Veeck L L, Hughes M, Rosenwaks Z 1999 First unaffected pregnancy using preimplantation; genetic diagnosis for sickle cell anaemia. Journal of the American Medical Association 281(18): 1701–1706

Yaish H M 2005 Thalassaemia. School of Medicine, Department of Pediatrics, Utah University of Utah. Online. Available at: http//www.emedicine.com

Chapter 6

Asthma

INTRODUCTION

Asthma is a common disorder of the respiratory system affecting more than 5 million people in the UK (NAC 2001). Although deaths have been declining steadily, asthma still causes much unnecessary suffering for patients. Overall however, asthma care is greatly improved due to significant improvements in treatment.

In asthma, the airways are narrowed after exposure to a trigger or an allergen causing difficulty in breathing. In many people, treatment with an inhaler and/or systemic drugs will keep this condition under control allowing them a normal, active life span. Stress is one of the factors that can aggravate asthma, and pregnancy and childbirth, causing both physiological and psychological stress, may result in a worsening of the condition. It is essential therefore that the midwife has a good understanding of this common condition to prevent asthma complicating the childbearing process.

RELEVANT ANATOMY AND PHYSIOLOGY

The respiratory system is responsible for providing oxygen to body cells to enable metabolism to take place. It is also responsible for removing carbon dioxide, which is the main waste product of this process. The cardiovascular system is closely associated with this function, as blood is the means by

Box 6.1 Homeostasis

Homeostasis is a condition in which the body's internal environment remains within certain physiological limits. For body organs and tissues to function efficiently, the composition of surrounding fluids must be precisely maintained at all times. Three factors are involved in maintaining homeostasis:

1. The optimum concentration of gases, nutrients, ions and water
2. An optimum body temperature
3. The correct volume of fluids within each fluid compartment.

Disturbance in homeostasis must be corrected quickly or illness may result. The body is constantly making adjustments to the internal environment to ensure homeostasis.

In asthma, carbon dioxide is retained in the body. Normally a rise in carbon dioxide levels within the body results in an increase in respiratory rate to remove the excess. In asthma, movement of air into and out of the alveoli is inhibited and carbon dioxide cannot be removed by this route. An increase in carbon dioxide results in a build up of H^+ (hydrogen ions) in the blood and a decrease in pH – respiratory acidosis. This causes an imbalance in homeostasis and other mechanisms will attempt to correct the acid–base imbalance. Substances in the blood (buffers) will bind with the hydrogen ions but these will quickly be used up. The renal system will excrete H^+ but again this can only partially compensate for the respiratory problems. Normal blood pH should be between 7.35–7.45. A pH < 7.35 will depress the nervous system and prevent normal body function. A pH < 7 will seriously depress the nervous system; the individual will become comatose and die if the respiratory acidosis is not quickly corrected.

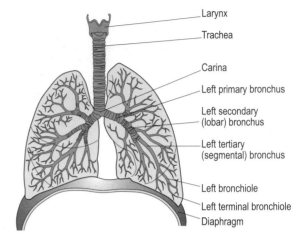

Figure 6.1   Organs and structures of the respiratory system.

which oxygen and carbon dioxide are transported to and from the cells. Any dysfunction of respiration (or circulation) will result in a disturbance of the homeostatic environment (Box 6.1), which is essential for cellular function. The relevant organs of the respiratory system are shown in Figure 6.1.

Ventilation

Respiration occurs by the inflation and deflation – ventilation – of the lungs. Air is thus taken into the alveoli of the lungs where gases are exchanged with the blood circulating in a capillary network surrounding these alveoli (Fig. 6.2). This occurs by simple diffusion across the membranes that separate the lumens of the alveolus and capillary (Fig. 6.3).

Inflation of the lungs – inspiration – is an active process; the muscles of the rib cage and diaphragm contract in response to nerve stimuli from the respiratory centre in the medulla of the brain. This causes the rib cage to enlarge and expand the lungs to which they are attached by membranes. Lung volume increases with a resultant decrease in pressure (Boyle's' Law). Air is drawn into the lungs down the pressure gradient, through the bronchi and bronchioles, to the alveoli where gases are exchanged as required.

Deflation of the lungs – expiration – is however a passive process. The muscles of the rib cage and diaphragm relax causing recoil of the elastic fibres of the lungs. Lung volume decreases and air is expelled. If there is excessive demand on the respiratory system, such as during exercise or breathing difficulties, the accessory muscles of respiration – those of the neck, shoulders and abdomen, become involved.

The amount of air moving into and out of the lungs in one ventilation is termed the tidal volume. With changing demand for oxygen and the removal of carbon dioxide, tidal volume is altered by an increase or decrease in ventilation rate and depth.

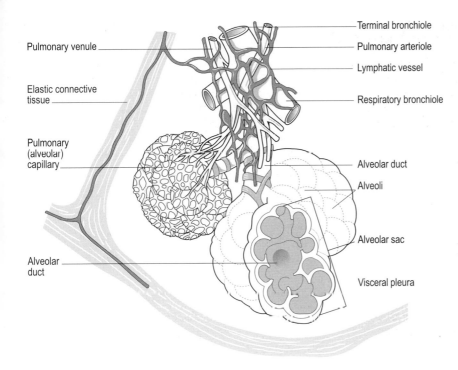

Pulmonary venule

Elastic connective tissue

Pulmonary (alveolar) capillary

Alveolar duct

Terminal bronchiole

Pulmonary arteriole

Lymphatic vessel

Respiratory bronchiole

Alveolar duct

Alveoli

Alveolar sac

Visceral pleura

Figure 6.2   Capillary network surrounding the alveoli.

Control of ventilation

Control of ventilation is normally involuntary. Voluntary control occurs to enable speaking or singing or, for example when swimming underwater or entering a smoke filled room. However, voluntary control is limited if homeostasis is severely threatened.

Ventilation is controlled by nerve cells in the respiratory centre in the brain stem. These receive input from chemoreceptors in the brain stem (bathed in cerebrospinal fluid) and in the aorta and carotid arteries. The composition of both cerebrospinal fluid (CSF) and blood reflect the levels of carbon dioxide (pCO_2) in the body. Chemoreceptors respond very quickly to any rise in pCO_2 by increasing the rate and depth of respiration. Thus, the respiratory system is able to rapidly respond to the needs of cells and ultimately of the body as a whole.

Factors that influence ventilation:

• Elasticity: Lung tissue consists of elastic connective tissue which allows expansion and

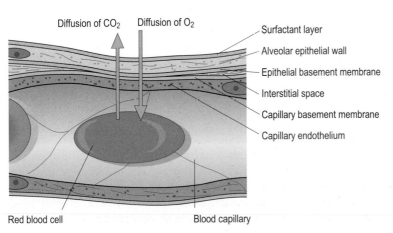

Diffusion of CO_2 Diffusion of O_2

Surfactant layer

Alveolar epithelial wall

Epithelial basement membrane

Interstitial space

Capillary basement membrane

Capillary endothelium

Red blood cell

Blood capillary

Figure 6.3   Diffusion of oxygen and carbon dioxide between capillary and alveoli.

contraction of lung size and volume. Damage to this tissue may cause a loss in elasticity and will necessitate forced expiration and increased effort on inspiration

- Compliance: Alveoli collapse when deflated. Some effort is required to reinflate them and this is aided by the presence of surfactant and the elasticity of alveolar walls. Compliance is a measure of the effort required to inflate the lungs, i.e. the alveoli
- Airway resistance: The diameters of the bronchi and bronchioles affect the volume of air that can move into and out of the lungs. If the airways are constricted by, for example bronchoconstriction (as in asthma), more effort is required to inflate the lungs.

ASTHMA

Asthma is a chronic inflammatory disease of the airways of the lungs. It is a common condition which is increasing in prevalence around the world (Rees & Kanabar 2000). The term 'asthma' comes from an ancient Greek word meaning 'panting'. The airways become narrowed and inflamed as a result of an inhaled allergen or trigger resulting in cough, wheeze and dyspnoea. An acute asthmatic attack can range in severity from mild shortness of breath to respiratory failure and death (Gutierrez & Peterson 2002). The alveoli themselves are not involved.

Asthma is thought to occur in 15% of children and 6% of adults in the UK (NAC 2001). Asthma that develops in childhood is usually provoked by an identifiable trigger, such as an allergen or by exercise. This is known as extrinsic asthma (Rees & Kanabar 2000). When asthma first develops in adult life, there is often no obvious stimulus other than respiratory tract infection – intrinsic asthma (Box 6.2). Many asthma sufferers however do not fit into either category.

Asthma is commonly considered to go through two primary stages: *hyperreactivity* and *inflammation*.

- In the *hyperreactivity* response, smooth muscles in the airways constrict and narrow inappropriately in response to an inhaled allergen. This is a normal protective reaction of the

Box 6.2 Occupational asthma

At least 1 in 10 cases of new or recurrent asthma in adults are caused by exposure to substances at work (McDonald 2005). There are many known substances that cause occupational asthma, including isocyanates that are found in many paints, flour and grain dust, animals and latex. Latex is a common product in use in the health services and latex allergies are becoming more common among midwives, as they have regular and prolonged exposure to the substance, mostly in examination gloves. Between 4% and 15% of healthcare workers have a reaction to latex, although this is usually contact dermatitis.

The risk of developing occupational asthma is connected to the level of exposure to the trigger and therefore, where possible, removing or reducing exposure will reduce the likelihood of developing a severe form of the disease.

respiratory system but the healthy person is able to breathe deeply and relax the airways to get rid of the allergen or irritant. In the asthmatic, the muscles of the airway do not relax and thus prevent deep breathing

- Subsequently, in the asthmatic, the immune system responds to the allergen by triggering the *inflammatory* response. White blood cells and other immune factors are delivered to the airways. These factors cause the airways to swell, fill with fluid and produce thick sticky mucus. This results in wheeze, breathlessness, inability to exhale adequately and a productive cough. The alveoli of the lungs stay partially inflated preventing sufficient fresh air, and therefore oxygen, from filling them. Effective diffusion of oxygen and carbon dioxide is thus prevented stimulating the asthmatic to increase ventilation depth and speed.

Causes of asthma

The incidence of asthma has risen dramatically worldwide over the past few decades and the reason for this is unclear. Many asthma sufferers also have allergies, but not all people with allergies have asthma. Some forms of asthma do not have an allergic trigger. Evidence to date suggests that asthma is due to a genetic susceptibility along with a variety of environmental triggers such as infection, diet, pollution and allergens (Siddall 2001). There is some evidence to implicate the overuse of antibiotics in early life with the increase in childhood asthma (Shirakawa et al 1997).

Pathophysiology of asthma

Asthma is caused by overactivity of the inflammatory response as a result of exposure to an allergen or trigger. Helper T cells overproduce a group of immune factors called interleukins which stimulate the production and release of antibodies known as immunoglobulin E (IgE). These IgE antibodies bind to mast cells found predominately in the lungs, skin and mucous membranes. In the lungs, mast cells release chemicals such as histamine, prostaglandins and thromboxane A_2. These result in spasm of the airways and the production of mucus. The presence of interleukins attracts leucocytes, specifically eosinophils, T lymphocytes and platelets, which accumulate in the airways. These remain in the airways for some weeks causing a late phase inflammatory response.

Repeated exposure to an allergen and the initiation of the above process causes permanent pathological changes to the structure and function of the airways resulting in chronic asthma (Fig. 6.4). The epithelial lining of the airways become thinned or destroyed causing increased sensitivity to the allergen on subsequent exposure. The damaged basement membrane of the epithelial layer is replaced with collagen and thus becomes less elastic preventing the airways from responding to the body's respiratory demands.

A person having an asthma attack is unable to expire effectively. As inspiration is an active process, the lungs are expanded by the contraction of the muscles of the rib cage and air will enter the lungs even when the airways are narrowed. However, expiration is a passive process; the intercostals muscles and diaphragm relax and air is expelled from the lungs.

When the airways are narrowed by the effects of asthma, the passage of air is restricted by the narrowed airways. The lungs are not sufficiently emptied and with the next inspiration, only a limited supply of fresh air (and oxygen) can enter. The pressure gradients of gases that enable diffusion of oxygen and carbon dioxide across the walls of the alveoli are lower; insufficient oxygen is supplied to the body cells and there is a rise in carbon dioxide in the blood. This is detected by chemoreceptors which signal the respiratory centre to increase the rate and depth of ventilation.

This does not solve the problem however. The narrowed airways prevent adequate movement of air out of the lungs however fast the person breathes. Body cells continue to be deprived of oxygen and also suffer from the build up of carbon dioxide causing a respiratory acidosis. Over time, the body cells will be unable to carry out necessary metabolic processes and the individual can become seriously ill. If not quickly treated,

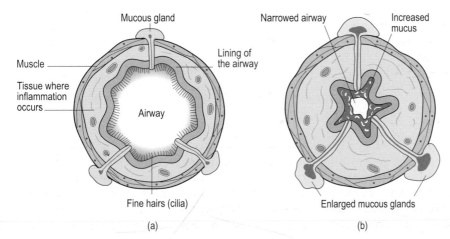

Figure 6.4   Changes to the airway in asthma. (a) Normal structure. (b) Structure in asthma.

Mucous gland

Lining of the airway

Muscle

Tissue where inflammation occurs

Airway

Fine hairs (cilia)

(a)

Narrowed airway

Increased mucus

Enlarged mucous glands

(b)

the individual will become exhausted with the increased respiratory effort; cells and organs will stop functioning due to lack of oxygen and death may occur.

Signs and symptoms

After exposure to a trigger, the classic asthmatic attack generally develops slowly over a few hours or days. In the majority of asthmatics, the attack occurs at night. Initially the patient begins to wheeze and experience dyspnoea and, if the attack becomes severe, the auxiliary muscles of respiration (shoulder, neck and abdomen) become active. Talking becomes difficult or impossible. Irritation of the nose (sneezing) and throat (cough), thirst and the need to urinate are common early symptoms. Mild to severe chest pain occurs in the majority of asthmatics and its intensity is unrelated to the severity of the attack. Once the attack ends, the asthmatic may develop a productive cough, with thick, stringy mucus. Inflammation of the airways persists for days or weeks after the attack, without symptoms, but must be treated to prevent a further asthmatic attack.

Asthma symptoms vary in intensity from occasional mild bouts of breathlessness to daily wheezing that persists, despite treatment. Asthma can be debilitating and frightening. Sleeplessness is a common problem.

Between 30–40% of women experience fluctuations in severity associated with their menstrual cycle, which are levelled out by the use of the oral contraceptive suggesting that hormones may have an effect on the condition (Ostrom 2006).

Diagnosis

A full medical history is taken including the circumstances surrounding the onset of symptoms, such as respiratory infection, exposure to cold, time of the year (spring is a time of increased allergic triggers) or exercise. Family history is also important as there is a genetic component to the disease. Other diseases are considered with similar symptoms, such as upper respiratory tract infection.

Lung function tests will confirm the diagnosis and determine the severity of the disease. A spirometer measures the volume of air inhaled and exhaled from the lungs. Two measurements are of particular relevance in asthma:

1. Peak expiratory flow rate (PEFR): This is the maximum flow rate that can be produced during a forced exhalation.
2. Forced expiratory volume (FEV1): This is the maximum volume of air forcibly expired in one second.

During an asthmatic attack, narrowing of the airways will result in a decrease in both of the above measurements. After treatment with a bronchodilator, an improvement in the measurements will confirm the diagnosis of asthma.

Laboratory tests may include skin and blood allergy tests if a specific allergen is suspected and examination of sputum may show increased levels of eosinophils and other leucocytes confirming an allergic cause of asthma.

Treatment

Monitoring the symptoms, avoidance of possible allergens and drug therapy will minimize the debilitating effects of asthma and prevent acute attacks. Control of asthma is aimed at attaining minimal chronic symptoms, minimal exacerbations, minimal emergency visits to medical services and no limitations on activity.

Self-monitoring A peak flowmeter is the standard monitoring device. In mild to moderate asthma, a single recorded morning measurement will give a good indication of any worsening of the condition. In severe asthma, this measurement may be required 2–3 times/day. The asthmatic will also be asked to record attacks, exposure to known allergens or triggers and medications taken.

Avoidance of possible allergens If the causative allergen or trigger can be identified, it may possibly be avoided, reducing the frequency of acute asthmatic attacks. Often however, this necessitates considerable modification of the home or work environment. House dust mites are often implicated in asthma and removal of soft furnishings; covering mattresses with an impermeable hypoallergenic material; and replacement of down pillows may be required. Pet hair may be a trigger and therefore keeping pets should be discouraged.

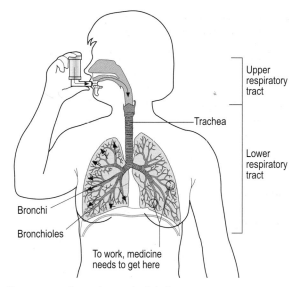

Upper
respiratory
tract

— Trachea

Lower
respiratory
tract

Bronchi

Bronchioles

To work, medicine
needs to get here

Figure 6.5   Drug therapy by inhaler.

Smoking cessation is an important area of lifestyle change and the asthma sufferer should be offered support and counselling to achieve this.

Research indicates that insufficient education of the asthmatic is often the cause of deterioration of the condition (Holmes 2002). Careful instruction and observation of the use of the inhaler and the peak flowmeter are vital in the treatment of asthma. The increasing involvement of practice nurses in the monitoring of asthma allows more time to be spent educating the patient (Stevens 2003).

Drug therapy   Drug therapy consists of prevention of long-term persistent inflammation and relief of acute symptoms. Drug therapy is best delivered by inhalation (Fig. 6.5) and >90% of asthma sufferers have no requirement for other methods of drug administration (Jordan 2003). Drugs that may be used to reduce inflammation include corticosteroids, leukotriene agonists and chromones.

Corticosteroids   Corticosteroids are powerful antiinflammatory drugs. They reduce inflammation and hence reduce oedema and secretion of mucus into the airway. These can be taken by inhalation or systemically. Inhalation of steroids by metered dose inhaler ensures that there is effective local antiinflammatory action with minimal systemic effects. Low doses may be sufficient for those suffering from mild asthma. Some side-effects may be experienced, such as hoarseness and dry throat. Oral steroids are used as a last resort, as they can cause serious side-effects. These are useful after an acute attack but only in severe cases are they used routinely. Side-effects when used long term are the development of conditions such as osteoporosis, diabetes and adrenal insufficiency. Inhaled corticosteroids include beclometasone, while prednisone or prednisolone are commonly used orally.

Leukotriene agonists   Leukotriene agonists act on the immune system preventing the damaging chemicals leukotrienes from causing inflammation and spasm of the airways. These drugs have a different action than corticosteroids and are thus useful in combination with steroids when asthma is not completely controlled by inhaled steroids alone. They are tolerated well and are especially useful in those with mild to moderate asthma (Coakley 2000). Very few side-effects have been identified other than gastrointestinal upset.

Chromones   Chromones, such as sodium cromoglicate, work both as an antiinflammatory and as a specific blocking agent for triggers such as allergens and exercise. Although only effective in 33% of asthma sufferers, these are useful drugs with few side-effects (Jordan 2003).

Control of acute symptoms is carried out by the use of bronchodilators. These include:

- $Beta_2$ adrenoreceptor agonists, such as salbutamol and rimiterol, which are given by inhaler or by nebulizer, depending on the individual's condition. These are effective for 3–6 h and relax smooth muscles to dilate the constricted airways. These drugs are only administered to relieve symptoms or as premedication for exercise induced asthma. Some side-effects may be experienced, such as anxiety, or a fast and irregular pulse
- Theophylline acts by relaxing the smooth muscles of the airways and also stimulates breathing. This drug is usually taken orally. Care must be taken to take the drug exactly as prescribed as overdosage can easily occur. Toxicity causes nausea and vomiting, headache and rarely, convulsions

- Anticholinergic drugs, such as ipratropium, act slowly to produce bronchodilation. These drugs are rarely used but may be useful if the asthmatic does not respond effectively to beta$_2$ agonists.

Prognosis Approximately 2000 people die in the UK each year from asthma. Most deaths occur in the elderly and are preventable. With effective treatment of asthma, it is very rare for someone to die of asthma. However, fatal or near fatal asthmatic attacks are commonly the result of underestimating the severity of the attack either by the asthmatic himself or the medical practitioner involved.

Asthma is a chronic condition, although some asthmatics experience long periods of remission. In mild to moderate cases, the condition may improve over time with effective treatment. With more severe cases, the structure and function of the airways are affected leading to irreversible changes in lung function.

Asthma causes considerable morbidity when symptoms persist resulting in loss of time from school and work. Sleep disturbances are common and can lead to poorer daytime performance (Rees & Kanabar 2000). A total of 46% of asthma sufferers report daytime symptoms; 30% asthma sleep related disturbances; and 25% require unscheduled urgent treatment indicating poor control of the condition.

ASTHMA IN PREGNANCY

Overview

The woman who presents with asthma in pregnancy can be affected in a number of ways. She may find her asthmatic condition is unaffected by her pregnancy, or the condition may be improved, or, in other instances, pregnancy may have an adverse affect on her asthmatic condition (SIGN 2004). She may rarely find that her condition seriously limits her normal activities (Beckman 2002). Poorly controlled asthma has been shown to be associated with adverse health outcomes in pregnant women, such as pregnancy-induced hypertension and pre-eclampsia, with associated interventions resulting from these conditions (Martel et al 2005). Women who have well-controlled asthma during pregnancy have outcomes comparable with non-asthmatic women.

Physiological changes in pregnancy

Pregnancy brings an increase of about 15% in metabolic rate due to anatomical and physiological changes in the female body and the presence of the fetus and placenta. There is therefore a greater demand for oxygen, of approximately 20%, and for the removal of carbon dioxide. Early in pregnancy, increasing levels of hormones, particularly progesterone, result in a considerable increase in tidal volume to enable these changes. There is normally no increase in ventilation rate.

Increased tidal volume is achieved by relaxation of the intercostal muscles, resulting in an increased transverse diameter in the rib cage of up to 2 cm. Additionally, the subcostal angle increases from 68° to 103° (Stables & Rankin 2005) and the diaphragm rises by an extra 4 cm (Fig. 6.6). Resultant tidal volume at rest increases from 500 mL to 700 mL during pregnancy.

The result of increased tidal volume is an overall decrease in pCO$_2$. This has little effect on the healthy pregnant woman but enhances the removal of carbon dioxide from the placenta and thus from the fetus.

The effect of progesterone is also seen on the smooth muscles of the bronchioles. Airway resistance is reduced and enables greater air flow into

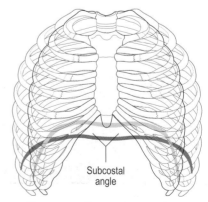

Subcostal angle

Figure 6.6   Changes to rib cage in pregnancy.

the lungs with decreased effort. This is countered later in pregnancy by the enlarging uterus pressing up on the base of the lungs, sometimes resulting in a degree of dyspnoea.

Incidence

The incidence of asthma in the general population is increasing and thus occurs in 1–2% of pregnant women (Tan & Thomson 2000). As with the general population, the prevalence of asthma is increasing in the population of childbearing women, making asthma the most common pre-existing medical disorder encountered in pregnancy. Management therefore, must be meticulous, and changes in treatment must be fully discussed with the woman in order to gain her cooperation.

Management of asthma in pregnancy

The management of moderate to severe asthma requires a cooperative approach between obstetricians, physicians, midwives, physiotherapists and the woman concerned. The aim of treatment is to optimize asthma management and client education and self-management plans are invaluable in achieving good outcomes.

The British Asthma Guidelines (BTS & SIGN 2004) provide a stepwise approach to asthma management (Fig. 6.7) and focus on the client being symptom free both day and night and on preventing acute attacks. The guidelines recommend that drug treatment of asthma in pregnancy is similar to that of the non-pregnant woman. Minimal drugs should be used to achieve good control of the condition.

Step 5:	Continuous or frequent use of oral steroids
Step 4:	Persistent poor control
Step 3:	Add-on therapy
Step 2:	Regular preventer therapy
Step 1:	Mild intermittent asthma

British Asthma Guidelines 2003

Figure 6.7 Stepwise approach to management of asthma.

All drugs commonly used to treat asthma, including short and long acting $beta_2$ agonists, inhaled corticosteroids, and oral and intravenous theophylline, are considered safe in pregnancy. Leukotriene receptor antagonists should not be commenced during pregnancy, but may be continued in women who, prior to pregnancy, have demonstrated significant improvement not achieved with other medications (SIGN 2004). Oral corticosteroids however, may increase the risk of congenital abnormalities such as cleft lip if taken in the first trimester (Park-Wyllie et al 2000). Intrauterine growth restriction and pre-term delivery are also associated with oral corticosteroids if taken over a long period in pregnancy (Bracken et al 2003). Evidence however, suggests that it is safer for the pregnant woman with asthma and her unborn child to be treated adequately than to have asthma symptoms or exacerbations (NAEPP 2005). Therefore, repeated reassurance must be given regarding the importance and relative safety of medication to ensure compliance.

The British Asthma Guidelines (BTS & SIGN 2004) also recommend offering advice on non-pharmacological control of asthma, by avoiding pollutants, such as car exhaust fumes, house dust mite, smoke inhalation and suggesting breathing exercises, acupuncture, hypnosis or yoga, to suit the individual woman. Beneficial effects of these non-pharmacological measures have not been proven.

Midwifery management

Midwifery care during pregnancy of the woman with asthma is similar to that of any pregnant woman and should take account of physical, psychological, social and educational factors.

The woman with established asthma often has a good working knowledge of her condition and the role of the midwife is to act as a facilitator if she requires help from other agencies. The newly diagnosed woman will, in addition, require support and guidance at her level of understanding.

Pre-pregnancy Ideally, women with asthma should be offered or seek pre-pregnancy counselling; this will allow a full history to be obtained and discussion of concerns will enable the woman to voice her anxieties. The health professional will discuss diet, contraception and smoking cessation and provide general health information, stressing the importance of continuing asthma medication during pregnancy to ensure good asthma control. Smoking cessation is strongly promoted, as maternal smoking during pregnancy is known to be associated with childhood asthma (Li et al 2005).

Many women are concerned about the effects asthma medication may have on the fetus. A recent large study indicates that many women decrease or cease the use of asthma medications in early pregnancy (Enrique et al 2006). Most asthma medication is safe to continue during pregnancy, but the woman must be referred to a registered medical practitioner for review (NMC 2004). Unfortunately, pre-pregnancy counselling is not always available or taken up by those most in need.

Pregnancy   There is a clear role for the midwife in any complication relating to pregnancy. At the initial visit, a careful history of previous and present pregnancies, obtained in a systematic unhurried manner, will elicit accurate and relevant information. If asthma is suspected, the midwife should refer the woman to a registered medical practitioner for appropriate management. Pregnancy is a favourable time to review the patient's basic understanding of asthma and its management, including trigger avoidance, control, use of devices and medication. A personal action plan can be developed (Rey & Boulet 2007).

Documentation of both baseline observations and a detailed history is of paramount importance, as these will provide a basis for subsequent management. Baseline observations should include blood pressure, pulse, temperature and urinalysis.

A detailed history should include clinical features, which the woman may experience, such as a cough, which may or may not be spasmodic; complaints of chest tightness or discomfort; dyspnoea; and audible expiratory wheezing.

The midwife should also ascertain, through sensitive questioning, whether the asthma restricts the woman's normal activities or causes her to become easily tired; whether there are factors that trigger the onset of acute asthma; what exercise she takes (if any); and whether she takes her medication regularly as prescribed. The midwife

should also determine how often she uses rescue medication during acute exacerbations.

Management of acute asthma during pregnancy
The pregnant asthma sufferer may experience acute symptoms at any time throughout her pregnancy but a large study found that the most severe symptoms were likely to occur between 24–36 weeks of pregnancy (Bracken 2003). Signs of acute asthma include: increased respiratory rate >25/min, pulse >110/min, use of accessory muscles of respiration, an inability to complete a sentence in one breath and a 50% reduction in peak expiratory flow (normally 480 L/min). Treatment must be prompt and adequate to bring the attack under control, as the risk of harm to the fetus from hypoxia outweighs any small risk from the medications required (SIGN 2004).

Acute severe asthma during pregnancy is an emergency and should be treated vigorously in hospital. This is a life-threatening condition. The woman will present with cyanosis, feeble respiratory effort, exhaustion, confusion and bradycardia. Peak expiratory flow will be <33% of the norm.

Principles of care:

- Obtain obstetric and medical aid
- Pulse oximetry – if SaO_2 <92% or if life-threatening features are present, the physician may order measurement of arterial gases
- Humidified oxygen therapy should be commenced to maintain saturation above 95%
- Secure venous blood samples for full blood count, urea and electrolytes and blood glucose
- Commence i.v. fluids, e.g. normal saline 8-hourly
- Give drug therapy for acute asthma as for the non-pregnant woman
- Position upright with a table to lean on, as this allows the accessory muscles to aid respiration
- Provide support and information
- Continuous monitoring of fetal heart by cardiotocography
- Documentation of all care including drugs administered should be recorded timeously and accurately
- Delivery should be considered and preparations made.

Labour and birth   Research indicates that symptoms decrease significantly in the last 4 weeks of pregnancy and 90% of pregnant women have no asthma symptoms during labour or birth (Nelson-Piercy 2001). Providing a calm environment, competent knowledge and continuity of care by the midwife can do much to foster the well-being of both woman and fetus. Progress during labour must, as ever, be recorded accurately. Women should continue their asthma medications. Women who are prescribed oral corticosteroids, such as prednisolone at a dose >7.5 mg/day for more than 2 weeks prior to labour, should be prescribed parenteral hydrocortisone 100 mg 6–8-hourly during labour until they can restart their oral medication (SIGN 2004). Where symptoms of acute asthma occur, medical assistance should be obtained promptly.

Asthmatic women may safely use all forms of pain relief in labour including epidural analgesia and Entonox, although if the woman has had recent acute asthmatic attacks, opioids such as pethidine and morphine should be avoided. These drugs stimulate the release of histamine, which causes bronchospasm and may trigger an acute asthmatic attack. Epidural anaesthesia is a good choice, as it reduces bronchospasm (Rey & Boulet 2007). Syntocinon is used in preference to Syntometrine or ergometrine in active management of the third stage, as ergometrine has been found to cause bronchospasm.

Management of the puerperium   Care in the puerperium of the mother with asthma will not differ from normal midwifery management. However, particular attention should be paid to the prevention of infection in the woman who is on oral corticosteroids, as she may be immunocompromised by the action of these drugs.

Breast-feeding is recommended to all women but exclusive breast-feeding has distinct advantages in the baby of the mother with asthma, as it is thought to reduce the incidence of the infant developing asthma (Kull et al 2002, Oddy et al 2004).

There is no evidence that drugs used routinely in the treatment of asthma are harmful to the breast-fed infant.

Baby of a mother with asthma   The development of asthma has both genetic and environmental components. The baby of a woman with asthma is therefore at increased risk of developing asthma. Breast-feeding confers some protection against this. However, there is a growing body of evidence to suggest that the fetus becomes sensitized to allergens in utero, with some infants showing raised IgE levels in cord blood at birth (Warner 2004). Other studies have shown an increase in asthma associated with some maternal occupations (Magnusson et al 2006) or a low maternal intake of vitamin E intake during pregnancy (Devereux et al 2006).

Future pregnancies   Asthma will follow a similar course in subsequent pregnancies. Therefore, the midwife can usefully emphasize to the mother in the puerperium the advantages of attending for pre-conception counselling. Thus, the woman will be able to achieve optimum health and optimal control of her asthma before embarking on another pregnancy.

A useful support group for parents and other sufferers of asthma is www.asthma.org.uk

REFERENCES

Beckman C A 2002 Descriptive study of women's perceptions of their asthma during pregnancy. American Journal of Maternal and Child Nursing 27:98–102

Bracken M B, Triche E W, Belanger K et al 2003 Asthma symptoms, severity and drug therapy: a prospective study of effects on 2205 pregnancies. Obstetrics and Gynecology 102:739–752

British Thoracic Society (BTS) Scottish Collegiate Guideline Network (SIGN) 2004 British Guidelines on the Management of Asthma. SIGN, Edinburgh

Coakley A 2000 Leukotrienes: new therapies and their influence on asthma. British Journal of Nursing 9(12):750–754

Devereux G, Turner S W, Craig L C A et al 2006 Low maternal vitamin E intake during pregnancy is associated with asthma in 5 year old children. American Journal of Respiratory and Critical Care Medicine 174(5):499–507

Enrique R, Pingshang W, Griffin M R et al 2006 Cessation of asthma medication in early pregnancy. American Journal of Obstetrics and Gynecology 195:149–153

Gutierrez K J, Peterson P G 2002 Pathophysiology. WB Saunders, Philadelphia

Holmes B 2002 Dual therapy for asthma comes of age. Practice Nursing 13(1):36–39

Jordan S 2003 Pharmacology for midwives. Houndmills, Palgrave

Kull I, Wickman M, Lilja G 2002 Breast feeding and allergic diseases in infants – a prospective birth cohort study. Archives of Diseases in Childhood 87(6):478–481

Li Y F, Langholz B, Salam M T 2005 Maternal and grandmaternal smoking patterns are associated with early childhood asthma. Chest 127(4):1232–1241

Magnusson L L, Wennborg H, Bonde J P, Olsen J 2006 Wheezing, asthma, hay fever and atopic eczema in relation to maternal occupations in pregnancy. Occupational and Environmental Medicine 63(9):640–646

Martel M J, Rey E, Beauchesne M F et al 2005 Use of inhaled corticosteroids during pregnancy and risk of pregnancy induced hypertension: nested case-control study. British Medical Journal 330(7485):230–233

McDonald J C 2005 Incidence by occupation and industry of acute work related respiratory disease in the UK, 1992–2001. Occupational and Environmental Medicine 62(12):836–842

NAC 2001 Out in the open. Asthma Journal 6(Suppl 3): 1–14

NAEPP 2005 Managing asthma during pregnancy; recommendations for pharmacologic treatment – 2004 update. NAEPP Expert panel report. Journal of Allergy and Clinical Immunology 115:34–46

Nelson-Piercy C 2001 Asthma in pregnancy. Thorax 56(1):325

Nursing and Midwifery Council 2004 Midwives rules and standards. NMC, London

Oddy W H, Sherriff J L, de Klerk N H 2004 The relation of breastfeeding and body mass index to asthma and atopy in children: a prospective cohort study to age 6 years. American Journal of Public Health 94(9):1531–1537

Ostrom N K 2006 Women with asthma: a review of potential variables and preferred medical management. Annals of Allergy, Asthma and Immunology 96(5):655–665

Park-Wyllie L, Mazzotta P, Pastusak A et al 2000 Birth defects after maternal exposure to corticosteroids; prospective cohort study and meta analysis of epidemiological studies. Teratology 62:385–392

Rees J, Kanabar D 2000 ABC of asthma. BMJ Books, London

Rey E, Boulet L 2007 Asthma in pregnancy. British Medical Journal 334(7593):582–585

Scottish Intercollegiate Guidelines Network (SIGN) 2004 British guidelines on the management of asthma. SIGN, Edinburgh

Shirakawa T, Enomoto T, Shimazu S I, Hopkin J M 1997 The inverse association between tuberculin responses and atopic disorder. Science 275:77–79

Siddall R 2001 Atopic asthma and allergen avoidance. Practice Nursing 12(6):217–219

Stables D, Rankin J (eds) 2005 Physiology in childbearing, 2nd edn. Elsevier, Edinburgh

Stevens N 2003 Inhaler devices for asthma and COPD: choice and techniques. Professional Nurse 18(11):641–645

Tan K S, Thomson N C 2000 Asthma in pregnancy. American Journal of Medicine 109:727–733

Warner J O 2004 The early life origins of asthma and related allergic disorders. Archives of Diseases in Childhood 89(2):97–102

Chapter 7

Renal disorders

CHAPTER CONTENTS

INTRODUCTION

Urinary tract infections are much more common in women than men. One of the main reasons for this is the comparatively short urethra. Poor hygiene and sexual intercourse can both result in ascending infection from a contaminated perineum. The causative organisms are commonly of gastrointestinal origin. In pregnancy, this is aggravated by the mechanical pressure of the enlarging uterus on the renal system and the relaxing effect of the hormones on the smooth muscles of the urinary tract.

Additionally, the kidneys can be compromised before a pregnancy even begins. Recurrent infections or other disease processes can both affect renal function. Major pathophysiological events during the childbearing process, such as haemorrhagic or endotoxic shock can also result in renal disease or failure. The midwife must be able to recognize signs of renal compromise and understand the effect this has on the childbearing process.

RELEVANT ANATOMY AND PHYSIOLOGY

The renal system is composed of (Fig. 7.1):

- Two kidneys, which produce urine
- Two ureters, which transport urine to the bladder
- The bladder, which stores urine and
- The urethra, which disposes of urine at a convenient time.

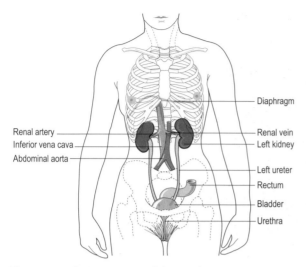

Figure 7.1   Gross structure of the renal system.

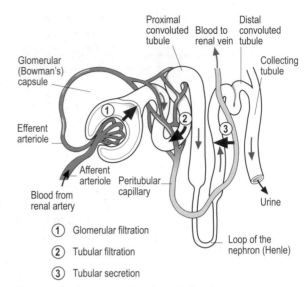

Figure 7.2   Structure of nephron indicating processes involved in urine production.

The kidney contains the functional units of the renal system – the nephrons. These microscopic structures, of which there are approximately 1 million, are responsible for several related functions. They filter and excrete water, electrolytes and nitrogenous waste products and maintain acid-base balance. They also play a major role in blood pressure control via the renin–angiotensin pathway, and produce erythropoietin factor, a substance involved in the production of red blood cells.

To achieve these major functions, the kidneys receive 20–25% of arterial blood directly from the aorta. The majority of this blood is transported directly to the nephrons where urine is produced. The anatomy of the nephron is shown in Figure 7.2. Three major processes are involved in urine production:

1. Glomerular filtration
2. Selective tubular absorption
3. Tubular secretion.

Glomerular filtration

Filtration is the process by which water and dissolved substances move across a membrane under pressure. The afferent arteriole of the Bowman's capsule has a comparatively larger diameter than the efferent arteriole which leads away from the capsule. This anatomical arrangement produces an increased pressure in the capillaries contained within the glomerulus thus providing the pressure

required to drive filtration. Approximately 10% of the blood entering the glomerulus is filtered including the majority of the components of blood. Only those substances which are too large to pass through the walls of the capsule and capillaries, such as blood cells and proteins are normally retained in the circulating blood.

Net filtration pressure is the driving force of this process and is made up of three components: hydrostatic pressure in both the glomerular capillaries and Bowman's capsule, and osmotic pressure (Fig. 7.3). The filtrate that is produced is very dilute and contains both useful and waste products.

Selective tubular reabsorption

The second process reclaims substances useful or necessary to the body. Tubular reabsorption occurs along the length of the tubule of the nephron but there are three distinct sections that undertake different aspects of this process:

1. The proximal convoluted tubule reabsorbs water and solutes by both active and passive processes.
2. The loop of Henle passes through a concentration gradient which concentrates the urine without loss of valuable solutes.
3. The distal convoluted tubule further reabsorbs substances required by the body.

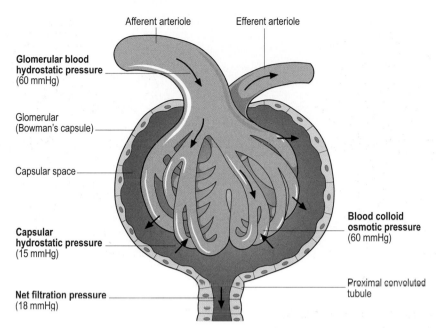

Afferent arteriole   Efferent arteriole

**Glomerular blood
hydrostatic pressure**
(60 mmHg)

Glomerular
(Bowman's capsule)

Capsular space

**Capsular
hydrostatic pressure**
(15 mmHg)

Net filtration pressure
(18 mmHg)

**Blood colloid
osmotic pressure**
(60 mmHg)

Proximal convoluted
tubule

Figure 7.3   Pressures involved in the process of filtration.

Tubular secretion

This third process is responsible for actively transporting substances from blood into the urine. Thus, excess hydrogen and potassium ions, and certain drugs that have escaped the filtration process are removed from the body. This process plays a vital role in acid-base balance.

Other functions of the nephron

Concentration of urine

The nephron is involved in several additional physiological processes. Fluid and electrolyte balance is achieved by the action of aldosterone and antidiuretic hormone. Aldosterone controls sodium reabsorption in the distal tubule. Antidiuretic hormone is responsible for the permeability of the distal tubule and collecting duct to water, and thus regulates the concentration of urine.

Blood pressure regulation

Another physiological process, in which the nephron plays a vital role, is in blood pressure regulation. Anatomically, the final section of the ascending limb of the loop of Henle comes into close proximity with the afferent arteriole of the nephron (Fig. 7.4). At this point, the walls of both

structures contain specialized cells forming the juxtaglomerular apparatus. The cells in the nephron make up the macula densa – a compact collection of cells that measure the amount of sodium in the filtrate. The corresponding cells in the arteriole, the juxtaglomerular cells, contain muscle fibres and granules of renin.

Renin is released into the bloodstream when the juxtaglomerular apparatus detects a decrease in circulating blood and/or decreased sodium levels in the glomerular filtrate. Renin reacts with an inactive fraction of plasma globulin, angiotensin I, which is then converted in the lungs into angiotensin II. This substance circulates in the blood acting on the smooth muscle of arterioles resulting in vasoconstriction. It also stimulates the secretion of aldosterone (thus retaining sodium in the kidneys) and to a lesser extent glucocorticoids. Glucocorticoids are involved in the production of glucose when blood sugar levels are low.

Manufacture of erythrocytes

Erythropoietin factor is produced in the kidneys. This substance is secreted into the bloodstream in response to hypoxia where it reacts with a plasma protein to produce erythropoietin. Erythropoietin stimulates the bone marrow to produce erythrocytes.

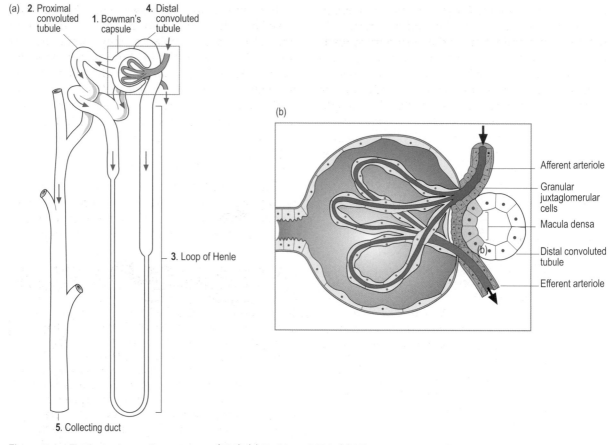

(a) 2. Proximal convoluted tubule 1. Bowman's capsule 4. Distal convoluted tubule

3. Loop of Henle

5. Collecting duct

(b)

Afferent arteriole

Granular juxtaglomerular cells

Macula densa

Distal convoluted tubule

Efferent arteriole

Figure 7.4   The juxtaglomerular apparatus (JGA). (a) Position of JGA. (b) Microstructure of JGA.

Synthesis of vitamin D

Calcitriol is activated in the kidneys. This substance is a component of vitamin D and requires conversion in the kidney to an active form before it can fulfil its role of stimulating calcium absorption in the gut.

Other structures of the renal system

Two ureters lead from the kidneys and drain urine into the bladder where it is stored. The bladder can hold approximately 600 mL but the desire to micturate is conveyed to the nervous system once 300 mL of urine is present. Finally, the urethra leaves the base of the bladder passing through the muscles of the perineum to the urethral orifice. As indicated above, the female urethra is considerably shorter than in the male which predisposes women to ascending urinary tract infections.

PATHOPHYSIOLOGY

Generally humans can survive with only one fully functional kidney. Only when disease processes damage a large proportion of the functional units, the nephrons, will renal function become impaired.

Disease processes of the renal system can be considered from two different aspects; infection of tissue with the potential for damage to the renal system, and actual damage to tissue from a disease process. For ease of understanding, pathophysiology will be discussed from these two viewpoints although it must be clearly understood by the midwife that each condition can lead to the other.

Aetiology

Infection

Bacteria from the gastrointestinal tract are the commonest causative agents in urinary tract infection. Often this is *Escherichia coli*. As a result of the close proximity of the urethral meatus to the anus, contamination of the perineum spreads easily into the urethra particularly if personal hygiene is poor. Abrasion of the urinary meatus during sexual intercourse can also result in entry of pathogens to the renal system. The short length of the urethra then enables infective organisms to reach the bladder easily and proliferate. Infection in the bladder may spread to the ureters and on into the kidney itself causing inflammation, pyelonephritis and possible damage to the nephrons themselves.

Chronic renal disease

Damage to renal tissue can be caused by a variety of events. Recurrent infections can lead to loss of functional tissue over time. Renal damage can occur secondary to another disorder, such as diabetes or hypertension. Structural defects of the renal system such as congenital abnormality or abnormalities such as tumours or polycystic kidneys will also cause long-term dysfunction. Glomerulonephritis is an autoimmune disease which may occur without obvious cause or secondary to a viral infection.

Acute renal failure

The kidneys are particularly vulnerable during any event where there is circulatory shut down (Perkins & Kisel 2005). Acute blood loss, toxic shock from overwhelming infection can both lead to acute renal failure as can a urinary obstruction or damage resulting in backflow of urine.

Pathophysiology

As already discussed, bacteria can enter the renal tract comparatively easily in women. Infection of the urinary tract will cause inflammation of affected tissues. Inflammation to the ureters, bladder and urethra will result in discomfort and pain. However, these structures are largely responsible for transport and storage of urine and thus inflammation will not have a major impact on renal function. If the infection reaches the kidneys however, this will result in disruption of the normal processes taking place in the nephrons.

Two important processes may be compromised by inflammation in the renal system. Fluid and electrolyte imbalance may occur as the inflamed tubules of the nephron become less efficient at reabsorbing sodium, which is then retained in body tissues and fluids. With retention of sodium, water is also retained, resulting in oedema and/or increased cardiac workload. Acid-base balance will also be affected as secretion of buffering substances is compromised and hydrogen ions are retained in the body (Box 7.1).

Chronic renal disease is usually the result of secondary damage to the kidneys as a result of another disease process. Commonly, this is due to hypertension but other causes are polycystic kidneys and

---

Box 7.1 Acid-base balance

Health and good body functioning are dependent both on fluid and electrolyte balance and acid-base balance. The renal system plays a vital role in the latter. Biochemical reactions in the cells of the body are very sensitive to even small changes in the pH of extracellular fluids (ECF). Normal pH of plasma and ECF is 7.35–7.45, which is slightly alkaline. Yet the foods and fluids we take into our bodies, and those present in some organs of the body, have a very different pH. Gastric juices in the stomach range from 1.2–3. Orange juice is 3.5; coffee is 5 and antacids 9–10.

The renal organs as well as other systems of the body therefore have the responsibility of maintaining the acid-base balance and the renal system is a vital part of this process.

Acid-base balance is maintained through three systems:

1. Buffering: A buffer is a chemical 'sponge' soaking up excess H^+ or releasing them. Examples of body buffers are bicarbonate, phosphate, proteins. Buffers work within a matter of seconds.
2. Respiration: Excess H^+ combine with other substances in the blood to produce CO_2, which is then excreted through an increase in ventilation rate. This process corrects imbalances in a matter of minutes.
3. The renal system acts over hours and days to stabilize a prolonged imbalance. The distal tubules remove excess H^+.

If there is renal dysfunction therefore, acid-base balance will be disturbed causing illness and potentially death.

glomerulonephritis. Examples of these related to pregnancy are:

- Diabetes in which the high level of circulating glucose encourages atherosclerosis resulting in diminished blood flow to the kidneys. The juxtaglomerular apparatus detects this, releases renin, vasoconstriction occurs and blood pressure rises. This further damages the glomerulus. Additionally, any infective organism given access to the renal system will proliferate in the tissues due to the increased glucose levels and this will further compromise the situation.

- Essential hypertension will result in increased blood pressure to the kidneys damaging the glomerular filtering membrane and allowing loss of protein into urine. Excretion of waste products will be inefficient and they will be found in increasing levels in the blood.

Whatever the cause of chronic renal disease, the inability to excrete metabolic waste and maintain fluid and electrolyte, and acid-base balance indicates a degree of renal failure. Homeostasis, the regulation of the internal environment to maintain a stable state, is disrupted and normal cell function is compromised. Waste products will build up in the blood – uraemia – and will lead to acidosis. As the condition worsens, other organs will become affected as the cells are unable to carry out their functions effectively. Blood pressure will rise in an attempt to move sufficient blood through the kidneys for the removal of the rising levels of wastes and excess electrolytes. This will further damage renal tissue.

Acute renal damage may occur as a result of a major pathophysiological crisis, such as haemorrhagic or toxic shock as described above. The nephrons in the kidney are starved of oxygen (ischaemia) and begin to die (necrosis). Other causes may be an acute infection as in pyelonephritis or an acute inflammation as in glomerulonephritis. Renal tissue is irritated by the causative organism or inflammatory process and is seriously damaged. An obstruction in the renal system resulting from renal stones (calculi) in the renal pelvis, ureters or bladder, will result in the accumulation of urine within the renal system

(Steggall 2001). This will cause increased pressure on all structures preventing normal function. In any of these events, the disruption is sudden and severe, and may result in acute renal failure. Renal function is severely compromised or ceases altogether and waste products accumulate in the bloodstream. The condition is however, usually reversible.

Signs and symptoms

Urinary tract infection is relatively common in women. Cystitis, infection or inflammation of the bladder, presents with frequency of urine, dysuria, urgency of micturition and suprapubic or lower back pain. If the infection spreads to the kidneys, pyelonephritis, these symptoms are accompanied by fever, nausea and vomiting, rigors and suprailiac pain.

Chronic renal disease is associated with generalized oedema and proteinuria. Other signs are hypertension and decreased urinary output. Serum urea and creatinine levels increase and may cause symptoms of confusion, malaise and apathy. Increased levels of these products in sweat may be indicated by skin irritation and itchiness.

Electrolyte imbalance will be demonstrated by symptoms associated with the related ion:

- Hyperkalaemia (high potassium levels) is associated with tachycardia/bradycardia with electrocardiogram changes, abdominal distension and diarrhoea. Hypokalaemia is associated with hypotension and cardiac dysrhythmias
- Hypernatraemia (high sodium levels) is associated with signs of dehydration, hypertension, tachycardia and oedema. Severe hypernatraemia can result in convulsions
- Hypercalcaemia (high calcium levels) causes muscle weakness, drowsiness and headache. Hypocalcaemia results in twitchiness, muscle spasm, numbness and irritability.

A corresponding metabolic acidosis may develop and will be demonstrated by low urinary and plasma pH, disorientation and shortness of breath or deep, rapid breathing.

Fluid imbalance will also be impaired and if severe, sudden onset of pulmonary oedema may occur. This will be indicated by symptoms of dyspnoea (shortness of breath), frothy sputum and decreased pO_2 levels.

With acute renal failure, many of the above signs and symptoms will appear over time but the first indication is likely to be oliguria (decreased urinary output <500 mL/day), which may progress rapidly to anuria (no urine output). The urine will contain blood as well as protein. As the condition worsens with severe fluid and electrolyte imbalance, the presence of abnormally high levels of waste products in the bloodstream may lead to disseminated intravascular coagulation.

Diagnosis

A range of diagnostic tests are available in the assessment of renal function.

Urinalysis

Urinalysis is relatively fast, simple and accurate and can give a good indication of renal function. Reagent strips enable the clinician to identify the presence of substances such as protein, glucose and blood, as well as measure pH and specific gravity (Box 7.2 on proteinuria). Both the appearance of the urine and its smell will give information regarding fluid balance and the presence of infective organisms.

Box 7.2 Proteinuria

Protein should never be present in urine. Protein molecules are too large to pass through the healthy glomerular filter in the nephron. Therefore, the presence of proteinuria always requires further investigation.

The first consideration however, must be whether the urine has been contaminated. This may be due to a dirty container for a sample of urine to be tested at the surgery. Alternatively, contamination may come from the vagina – an infection or discharge such as blood or liquor. A fresh mid-stream specimen of urine voided into a sterile container should prevent contamination. If proteinuria is still present, the urine will require laboratory analysis. Possible causes will be urinary tract infection or renal damage.

Bacteriological tests

Bacteriological culture of a clean catch fresh specimen of urine will identify the causative organism of a urinary tract infection. Sensitivity studies will determine the appropriate antibiotic to be used for treatment of the infection.

Biochemical tests

A 24-h collection of urine may be indicated when an accurate assessment of renal function is required. The total quantity of this substance, for example, protein or creatinine, allows calculation based on the person's height and weight and on the total quantity of urine excreted in that 24-h period. This allows a much more accurate determination of glomerular filtration than can be made on a single sample of urine.

Examination of the composition of blood is a vital indicator of renal function. Impaired glomerular function and loss of the ability of the tubules to reabsorb and secrete substances leads to increasing levels of waste products in the blood. The test commonly used to determine this is for urea and electrolytes. However, other blood tests can be ordered to look at the concentration of specific substances such as creatinine and urates.

Haematological tests can be ordered to consider such issues as white cell count, if infection is suspected, and haemoglobin levels. In cases of recurrent infection, anaemia is commonly also present.

Renal function tests

Two main types of tests are available which measure the function of either the glomerulus or the renal tubules. These are the two principal areas of renal function.

An estimation of glomerular function can be determined by looking at a substance that is normally freely filtered by the glomerulus and neither reabsorbed or secreted in the tubules. Creatinine is a waste product that is removed from the body by this process. A 24-h collection of urine for 'creatinine clearance' will give a clear indication of the efficiency of glomerular filtration, i.e. the glomerular filtration rate (GFR).

Tubular function is determined by considering its effectiveness at balancing water loss or retention. Antidiuretic hormone and aldosterone are released when whole body fluid volume or sodium levels are diminished. These act on the renal tubules which then reabsorb water and sodium respectively for retention in the body. If tubular function is compromised, this fine tuning of fluid balance is disrupted. The standard test for investigating tubule function is by estimating osmolality, the concentration of urine.

Other tests

A variety of other tests are now available to further investigate renal dysfunction:

- Radioisotope tests may be used to demonstrate renal dysfunction by labelling and measuring a substance normally excreted by the kidneys. An example of this test is ^{57}Cr-labelled EDTA
- Radioisotope scans follow the path of a substance as it passes through the renal system
- Ultrasound can look at the size and structure of the organs of the renal system and thus identify renal disease such as polycystic kidneys or the presence of tumours
- Intravenous pyelography is a procedure in which a radio-opaque dye is injected into the bloodstream and X-rays taken to view the structures of the renal system
- Cystoscopy involves the passage of a scope into the bladder via the urethra to visualize the internal surface of the bladder
- CT (computed tomography) or MRI (magnetic resonance imaging) can be used to detect tumours and cysts
- Renal angiography will examine the blood supply to the kidneys by following a radio-opaque dye through the blood vessels on X-ray. This will identify any stenosis of the vessels particularly of the renal artery leading into the renal system.

Treatment

Treatment of urinary tract infection is by the use of an appropriate antibiotic. Anaemia must also be treated if present, as this will predispose to recurrence of infection.

Chronic renal disease is managed conservatively as long as possible. If a treatable lesion has been identified, this may be surgically removed and renal function assessed and treated accordingly. The principles of management of renal disease are to prevent further deterioration if possible and to identify and treat any secondary damage to other organs or systems.

Diet, including fluid intake, is adjusted to minimize the production of waste and fluid. This usually entails a diet low in protein – <60 g/day – and an increase in carbohydrate to provide adequate calories (Fenglei et al 2005). Electrolytes are assessed and diet adjusted if required. Multivitamins and calcium are prescribed to replace dietary deficit.

Active management is required if these measures are insufficient to prevent life-threatening dysfunction of body organs and systems. *Peritoneal dialysis* or *haemodialysis* will be required until a kidney transplant can be arranged (Alonso et al 2005). Neither of these processes can totally replace normal renal function but will enable the patient to live a relatively normal life for some time. One of the essential functions of the kidney that cannot be replaced by dialysis is its endocrine function.

Acute renal failure is commonly a complication of another disorder and if treated promptly, is often reversible. Medical management is aimed at prompt recognition followed by commencement of dialysis to restore normal homeostasis and allow the return of normal tissue functioning.

THE RENAL SYSTEM IN PREGNANCY

Introduction

The renal system is affected in pregnancy both by the increase in circulating hormones and by the mechanical displacement associated with the gravid uterus. Women are particularly susceptible to urinary tract infection as a result and the midwife must be aware of this possibility when women present with lower back pain or proteinuria. Renal adaptation to pregnancy brings altered laboratory values and these must be appreciated when examining renal function. Should renal adaptation be coupled with pregnancy-induced complications or pre-existing renal dysfunction, renal function may be further compromised leading to an increased risk of maternal and fetal morbidity and mortality.

Physiological changes in pregnancy

During pregnancy, a number of changes take place as a result of the increasing levels of hormones. Renal blood flow increases by 70–80% (Thorsen & Poole 2002), peripheral resistance decreases and as a result, glomerular filtration increases by 30–50% (Gilbert & Harmon 1998). Waste products are therefore cleared from the body more effectively so that creatinine and urea levels are reduced in blood and increased in urine. Fluid and electrolyte balance is also affected by the increasing levels of hormones, particularly progesterone. Sodium is filtered at an increased rate and aldosterone levels increase to compensate. As a result, whole body sodium levels are higher and aid in the increased blood volume required for pregnancy. Additionally, glucose is lost more readily from the body as the renal threshold for glucose is exceeded. This last factor is one of the causes of the increased risk of urinary tract infection as glycosuria creates an ideal medium for bacterial growth (Lindheimer et al 2000).

The presence of the enlarging uterus also results in alteration of renal function. The effect of progesterone on the smooth muscle of the ureters and bladder especially on the right is aggravated by pressure from the uterus and urinary stasis increases the risks of ascending infection. From a more practical perspective, the pressure of the uterus on the bladder results in frequency of micturition early in pregnancy, while the uterus is enlarging in the pelvis and again towards the end of pregnancy when the head engages in the pelvis.

Incidence

Urinary tract infection is the most common infection experienced by women. It has been estimated that at least 50% of women will experience a urinary tract infection at some time in their lives (Bardsley 2003). The most common disease process related to pregnancy involving the renal system is infection. Up to 10% of pregnant women will develop a urinary tract infection. Acute renal failure is rare in pregnancy but must be considered in any sudden serious complication. Chronic disease is also rare but with an increasing number of women leaving pregnancy until later in life, renal disease may be a complication

of essential hypertension. An increasing number of women are also choosing pregnancy after renal transplantation (Yildirim & Uslu 2005).

Urinary tract infection

As described above, urinary tract infection is more common in woman and especially in women who are pregnant. Up to 10% of pregnant women have a high level of bacteria in their urine with no symptoms – asymptomatic bacteriuria (Lloyd 2003). If left untreated, 40% of these women will develop a urinary tract infection (UTI) and 30% of these, pyelonephritis.

Asymptomatic bacteriuria

Asymptomatic bacteriuria is a potentially harmful condition that many women demonstrate whether pregnant or not. Diagnosis is based on the presence of >100 000 bacteria/ml in a clean catch specimen of urine. A negative urinalysis for protein with dipstick is not a reliable indicator of absence of the condition in pregnant women (McNair et al 2000). All women should be screened for this condition therefore by laboratory analysis early in pregnancy and if present treated with antibiotics. A further specimen should then be tested to ensure effective treatment. Asymptomatic bacteriuria is associated with low birthweight babies, pre-term birth, hypertension, anaemia and pre-eclampsia (Samuels & Colombo 2002). Treatment with effective antibiotics has however shown a reduction in these risks (Smaill 2001). It has been suggested that asymptomatic bacteriuria may be associated more with deprivation and poor diet, which may predispose these women to both the condition and the above complications.

Cystitis

Symptomatic urinary tract infection complicates up to 3% of pregnancies. *Escherichia coli* is the most common organism seen with a symptomatic UTI and prompt treatment with antibiotics will reduce the risk of developing pyelonephritis (Vazquez & Villar 2003). If recurrent infections occur, further investigations should be carried out to rule out anaemia, which predisposes an individual to UTI particularly in pregnancy. Untreated symptomatic

UTI has been associated with congenital abnormalities, preterm birth, intrauterine growth restriction and intrauterine death (Samuels & Colombo 2002).

The presence of a UTI is usually suspected when the woman complains of frequency of micturition, dysuria and often lower back pain. Treatment is by broad spectrum antibiotic, considered safe for use in pregnancy.

Pyelonephritis

Acute pyelonephritis, which occurs in 1–2% of all pregnancies, is an important contributor to maternal morbidity. Pyelonephritis is commonly the result of an ascending untreated UTI and appears to be associated with pre-term labour.

The woman who develops acute pyelonephritis is generally very unwell. Signs and symptoms will include nausea and vomiting, extreme pyrexia, rigors and tachycardia. Lower abdominal pain may be accompanied with guarding. On examination, her urine will appear cloudy and smelly and demonstrate the presence of protein.

The woman with pyelonephritis will be admitted to hospital where she will be started on intravenous antibiotics. A broad spectrum antibiotic will be used initially and urine sent for urgent culture and sensitivity to ensure that this antibiotic is the appropriate one to use. This woman will require bed rest and an accurate record of her fluid intake and output to prevent dehydration from the effects of fever, nausea and vomiting if present. General midwifery care will include 4-hourly observations and the use of fans and tepid sponging to bring down fever. Abdominal examination should be carried out to identify the onset of pre-term labour. Thromboembolic complications will be prevented by the use of thrombo-embolism deterrent (TED) stockings and anticoagulant therapy (see Ch. 4).

After 48 h of intravenous antibiotics, oral medication will be commenced and continued for 14 days; the woman must be reminded of the importance of completing the course. Two weeks after completion a follow-up specimen of urine will be sent to the laboratory for culture, and monthly thereafter until birth. If a further UTI is diagnosed again in pregnancy, further investigations may be recommended postnatally.

Chronic renal disease

Chronic renal disease is often associated with infertility but with good medical care, and depending on the type and severity of the condition, women can successfully achieve a pregnancy with minimal fetal and maternal morbidity and mortality.

Pre-existing renal disease in pregnancy can present with generalized proteinuria and oedema, increased blood pressure and diminished urinary output. However, if well controlled, these symptoms rarely worsen in pregnancy unless hypertensive disorders of pregnancy are superimposed on impaired renal function (Gilbert & Harmon 1998). In this event, the compromised renal function may worsen into renal failure.

Treatment for chronic renal disease in pregnancy is complicated. Any hypertension must be controlled with antihypertensive drugs. Fluid and electrolyte balance will be closely monitored along with laboratory investigations of the excretion of waste products. An early 24-h urine sample will give a baseline against which the course of renal function can be measured. Diuretics may be used to aid excretion of retained fluids. Haemoglobin levels must be carefully monitored as pre-existing anaemia is likely, as the renal system has an important role in the production of erythropoietin. Added to this, the normal physiological haemodilution of pregnancy may lead to severe anaemia. Dietary advice and folic acid and iron supplementation may counter this to some degree.

Renal failure during pregnancy may require dialysis (Box 7.3). This carries a high fetal mortality rate (Davison 2001). However, recent advances in understanding and dealing with the complex pathophysiology has improved pregnancy outcome (Tan et al 2006).

Glomerulonephritis is unusual in pregnancy but if present, may mimic pre-eclampsia. In women with chronic glomerulonephritis there is an increased incidence of hypertension in later pregnancy but maternal and fetal outcomes are usually good (Fervenza et al 1997).

Acute renal failure

Acute renal failure in pregnancy is usually associated with a severe pregnancy-related event such as pre-eclampsia or haemorrhage. Infectious

Box 7.3 Renal dialysis

Renal dialysis is a form of renal replacement therapy, which provides an artificial replacement for lost kidney function due to acute or chronic renal failure. Dialysis is designed to support normal body function until renal recovery or until an alternative treatment can carried out such as renal transplant. Dialysis does not itself treat renal disease.

Dialysis is required to perform the two principal functions of the kidneys: waste and fluid removal. This is carried out by passing blood along one side of a semi-permeable membrane, while a dialysis solution flows by on the other side. High levels of wastes such as potassium and urea flow from the area of high concentration in the blood across the membrane into the dialysis solution, which is constantly replenished.

There are two main types of dialysis: haemodialysis in which the patient's blood is pumped into a dialyser for 3–4 h three times a week; and peritoneal dialysis, where a sterile solution is run into the patient's peritoneal cavity, left there for a period of time to absorb waste products and then removed.

causes include pyelonephritis, puerperal sepsis and septic abortion, whether induced or spontaneous. Rarely an unrelated accident such as trauma may result in acute renal failure. However, the incidence of acute renal failure in pregnancy has declined considerably with improved obstetric care and the use of aggressive antibiotic therapy.

Treatment in pregnancy follows the same path as for the general population, as discussed above. However, it will probably be advisable to terminate the pregnancy in acute renal failure, in the interest of the mother's condition.

Renal transplant

Pregnancy following renal transplantation is no longer uncommon (Lemini et al 2007). Women are however advised to refrain from pregnancy for 1–2 years after transplant. Immunosuppressants are considered safe for use in pregnancy and women must be advised to continue these as the risks of rejection outweigh fetal risks. Pre-eclampsia is not uncommon in these women but it can prove difficult to distinguish this from pre-existing hypertension and proteinuria.

Effect on fetal outcome

Maternal renal disease increases the incidence of fetal loss, intrauterine growth restriction and preterm birth. Maternal hypertension secondary to renal disease is the most common risk factor for adverse perinatal outcome (Sanders & Lucas 2001). The degree of maternal fluid and electrolyte imbalance is a crucial determinant of fetal compromise.

Throughout pregnancy, careful monitoring of fetal health and growth is essential to identify uteroplacental insufficiency and fetal hypoxia. Reduction in the glomerular filtration rate will allow higher concentrations of toxic substances and maternal drugs to cross the placental barrier and this must be considered when considering treatment options.

Midwife's management

Pregnancy

Ideally, any woman with pre-existing renal disease will be advised prior to conception of the risks to herself and the fetus. Advice can be given to achieve optimum health to minimize the additional risks to pregnancy outcome. A nutritious well-balanced diet will be advised where possible.

In pregnancy, women with renal disease will be monitored by the multidisciplinary team with increased frequency of visits to the midwife, obstetrician and nephrologist. Renal function will be assessed on a regular basis by examining haematological levels of urea and electrolytes. Urine samples will be tested for protein as well as glucose and blood. Where indicated, urine specimens will be cultured for infection and advice given regarding personal hygiene and recognition of UTI. The woman will be advised to seek early medical advice if she suspects she has developed an infection.

At each antenatal visit, the midwife should examine the woman closely for signs of superimposed hypertension or pre-eclampsia. Urinalysis and blood pressure measurement must be taken at every visit. Regular full blood counts will be undertaken to rule out anaemia or other complications of these conditions. Abdominal examination should be carried out and if there is any indication of slow fetal growth or diminished fetal movement, the midwife must arrange immediate medical review.

Admission to hospital for increased surveillance will be advised if either maternal or fetal condition deteriorates. Depending on gestation, the risk and benefits of continuing the pregnancy may need discussion.

In women with no previous history of renal disease, the midwife must be alert for any indication of urinary tract infection. Educating all women of the signs of UTI will enable infections to be treated promptly. Consideration must be made of the possible differential diagnoses of the cause of back pain, as the midwife should be aware of the risks of pre-term labour in women with a UTI. The midwife will advise the woman of the principles of good hygiene and of the value of drinking sufficient clear fluids daily (Turner 2000).

Labour

Labour and birth are a time of increased physiological and psychological stress for the woman at risk of complications. Women with renal disease will be strongly advised to give birth in a specialized maternity unit with intensive care facilities for both mother and baby. Labour will be managed by the obstetrician in close liaison with other relevant specialists. The midwife will care for this woman in a high dependency area where all facilities are available.

Puerperium

After the birth, care will continue in a high dependency area until the condition of both mother and baby is satisfactory. The midwife's role will be to carry out careful observations as instructed, including fluid and electrolyte balance. Because of the increased risk of acute renal failure, hourly urine measurement will be carried out.

Support and explanation to both the mother and her family will be a fundamental part of the midwife's role at this time. Caring for and feeding the baby will be difficult for this woman but the midwife must ensure that every opportunity is given to encourage mother and baby interaction.

Baby

The risks of pre-term labour and intrauterine growth restriction have already been discussed. The baby of a woman with renal disease is at increased risk of hypoxia and uteroplacental insufficiency. This baby therefore should be born in a unit with full neonatal intensive care facilities. Babies born to mothers who are on immunosuppressants for renal transplant will be more prone to infection as immunosuppressant therapy reduces the transmission of antibodies to the fetus (Lloyd 2003).

REFERENCES

Alonso A, Lau J, Jaber B L 2005 Biocompatible hemodialysis membranes for acute renal failure. Cochrane Database of Systematic Reviews. DOI: 10.1002/14651858. CD005283

Bardsley A 2003 Urinary tract infections: prevention and treatment of a common problem. Nurse Prescribing 1(4):114–117

Davison J M 2001 Renal disorders in pregnancy. Current Opinion in Obstetrics and Gynaecology 13:109–114

Fenglei X, Sumo M, Wu T 2005 Nutritional supplements for acute renal failure. Cochrane Database of Systematic Reviews. DOI: 10.1002/14651858. CD005426

Fervenza F, Green A, Lafayette R 1997 Acute renal failure due to postinfectious glomerulonephritis during pregnancy. American Journal of Kidney Disorders 29:273–276

Gilbert E S, Harmon J S 1998 Manual of High Risk Pregnancy and Delivery. Mosby, St Louis

Lemini M, Ochoa F, Gonzales M 2007 Perinatal outcome following renal transplantation. International Journal of Gynecology and Obstetrics 96(2):76–79

Lindheimer M, Grunfeld J, Davison J 2000 Renal disorders. In: Barron W, Lindheimer M, Davison J (eds) Medical disorders during pregnancy, 3rd edn. St. Louis, Mosby, p 39–70

Lloyd C 2003 Common medical disorders associated with pregnancy. In Fraser DM, Cooper MA (eds) Myles textbook for midwives, 14th edn. Churchill Livingstone, Edinburgh, p 321–356

McNair R D, MacDonald S R, Dooley S L, Peterson L R 2000 Evaluation of the centrifuged and Gram-stained smear, urinalysis, and reagent strip testing to detect asymptomatic bacteriuria in obstetric patients. American Journal of Obstetrics and Gynecology 182(5):1076–1079

Perkins C, Kisel M 2005 Utilising physiological knowledge to care for acute renal failure. British Journal of Nursing 14(14):768–773

Samuels P, Colombo D 2002 Renal disease. In: Gabbe S, Niebyl J, Simpson J (eds) Obstetrics: Normal and Problem Pregnancies. Churchill Livingstone, New York, p 1065–1080

Sanders C, Lucas M 2001 Renal disease in pregnancy. Obstetric and Gynecology Clinics of North America 28:593–600

Smaill F 2001 Antibiotics for asymptomatic bacteriuria in pregnancy. Cochrane Database of Systematic Reviews. Issue 2. Art No: CD000490. DOI: 10.1002/14651858 CD000490

Steggall M J 2001 Urinary tract stones: causes, complications and treatments. British Journal of Nursing 10(22):1453–1455

Tan L, Kanagalingam D, Tan H, Choong H 2006 Obstetric outcomes in women with end-stage renal failure requiring renal dialysis. International Journal of Gynecology and Obstetrics 94(1):17–22

Thorsen M S, Poole J H 2002 Renal disease in pregnancy. Journal of Perinatal & Neonatal Nursing 15(4):13–17

Turner 2000 How to manage urinary tract infections in pregnancy. British Journal of Midwifery 8(12):777–779

Vazquez J C, Villar J 2003 Treatments for symptomatic urinary tract infections during pregnancy Cochrane Database of Systematic Reviews. DOI: 10.1002/14651858. CD002256

Yildirim Y, Uslu A 2005 Pregnancy in patients with previous successful renal transplantation. International Journal of Gynecology and Obstetrics 90:198–200

Chapter 8

Epilepsy and other neurological conditions

CHAPTER CONTENTS

INTRODUCTION

Epilepsy is one of the most common neurological disorders seen in pregnant women. It is also responsible for increased maternal and fetal mortality and morbidity rates in the UK. In the most recent Confidential Enquiries into Maternal and Child Health 2000–2002 (Lewis & Drife 2004), there were 13 deaths from epilepsy during childbirth. Epilepsy is a disorder of the central nervous system in which neurons are inappropriately stimulated causing abnormal sensations and seizures. Other disorders of the nervous system that may be seen by the midwife are multiple sclerosis and myasthenia gravis, which will be briefly discussed at the end of the chapter.

Epilepsy is a condition in which nerve cells – neurons – are stimulated in a disorganized way, resulting in abnormal movements, such as fits, strange sensations, flashing lights, or smells that do not actually exist. Epilepsy occurs commonly in young people and therefore a midwife must understand the condition and its effects on pregnancy and childbirth.

The goal in caring for the pregnant woman with epilepsy is to keep her relatively free of seizures and to minimize the effects of epilepsy on both the pregnant woman and her fetus. Antiepileptic drugs can have a teratogenic effect on the fetus. During an epileptic fit, the woman may fall and injure herself or her baby, and may suffer from hypoxia, which could also affect the fetus. Knowledge of the condition, its signs and symptoms and how to prevent epileptic seizures by supporting women to comply with treatment, is essential in midwifery practice.

RELEVANT ANATOMY AND PHYSIOLOGY

The central nervous system is made up of the brain containing the cerebral cortex, which contains centres of motor and sensory control, and the spinal cord, through which nerve pathways carry neurons to all parts of the body (Fig. 8.1). Neurons detect changes in both the internal and external environment and respond to them to maintain homeostasis with body organs and systems. Epilepsy is an abnormal functioning of these neurons.

The cerebrum is composed of two cerebral hemispheres which are separated from each other, except at a point deep in the substance of the brain where a broad band of nerve fibres, the corpus callosum, enables communication between the two hemispheres. Each cerebral hemisphere is a mirror twin of the other and each has a complete set of centres responsible for sending, receiving and interpreting information. The cerebral hemispheres are responsible for the functions of the opposite side of the body but are capable of taking over some of the functions of the other hemisphere if the corresponding area has been damaged.

The central nervous system is composed of two principal types of tissue: grey matter which contains the cell bodies of neurons, and white matter through which neurons travel. The white

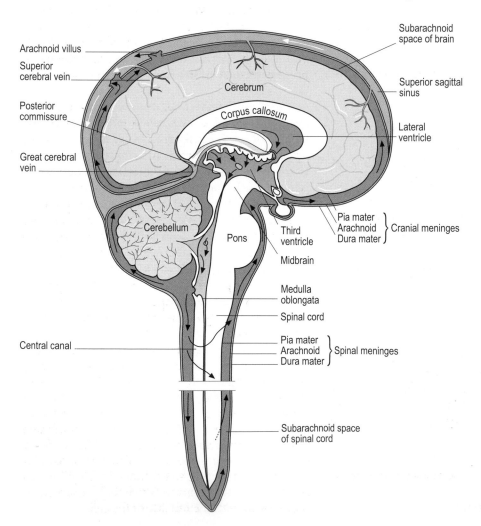

Figure 8.1 Gross structure of the central nervous system.

appearance is due to the colour of the myelin sheath that surrounds neurons (see below). Cell bodies appear grey as they are not surrounded by myelin.

In the cerebral cortex, the outer 2–4 mm of tissue contains cell bodies, appears grey and is known as the cerebral cortex. It is in this region of the brain where the majority of functional centres are situated and these interpret and act upon information received by the nervous system. The lighter 'white' matter of the brain fills the substance of the cerebrum. Interspersed throughout the white matter are other visible areas of grey matter known as nuclei, in which specialist interpretation of the environment is carried out.

In the spinal cord, the order of the white and grey matter is reversed, with white matter enclosing an H-shaped area of grey matter. This arrangement provides the cell bodies of neurons passing through the cord with maximum protection from injury. Once damaged, cell bodies cannot be repaired.

Other regions of the central nervous system include:

- The hypothalamus, which lies deep in the base of the cerebral hemispheres – this is linked to and controls the pituitary gland situated immediately below it. Through this relationship, it plays a major role in maintaining bodily homeostasis

- The medulla oblongata, which is situated just above the spinal cord and contains many vital centres that control such processes as cardiac and respiratory function

- The cerebellum, which projects posteriorly from the base of the cerebrum. This is concerned with learned patterns of movement, and with posture and balance.

The nervous system is made up of millions of small functional units called neurons supported by a network of specialist connective tissue called neuroglia. Neurons are cells that have been modified to transmit information in the form of an action impulse or electrical pulse between different parts of the body.

A neuron consists of (Fig. 8.2):

- A cell body containing the nucleus and other cell organelles
- An axon of varying length

- Dendrites that are stimulated by external factors
- Synaptic end bulbs, which transfer an action impulse to another neuron or structure, such as a muscle cell.

There are two principal types of neuron: those with a myelin sheath surrounding the axon and those without. Myelin is a fatty substance which insulates the axon from the surrounding environment preventing the loss of substances including ions which are responsible for the production of an action impulse. Neurons surrounded by myelin transmit an impulse much more quickly than those without: myelinated at on average of 120 m/s, unmyelinated at around 5–10 m/s.

The function of a neuron is to transmit information in the form of an action potential from one area to another. An action potential is a change in the electrical potential across the cell membrane of the neuron. This alters from -70 mV to $+35$ mV. This change in electrical potential is brought about by the movement of ions across the cell membrane.

Most cell membranes in the body maintain an electrical imbalance between the intracellular fluids within the cell and the extracellular fluids surrounding the cell. This is brought about by an imbalance in the concentration of potassium cations (K^+), sodium cations (Na^+) and associated anions. The fluids inside the cell contain an increased concentration of K^+ and a decreased concentration of Na^+. Those outside the cell have a decreased concentration of K^+ and an increased concentration of Na^+. This imbalance is maintained by a sodium potassium pump and by the greater permeability of the cell membrane to K^+ than to Na^+ and is called the resting potential of the cell membrane.

In the neuron, this imbalance is also present and is used to create a rapid change in electrical charge along the length of the axon (Fig. 8.3). As a result of stimulation of a dendrite (by a change in temperature, stretch in an organ, damage to cells for example), sodium channels in the cell membrane near to the dendrite open and allow Na^+ to flood into the cell. This process is called depolarization and the result is that the inside of the cell at this point on the axon becomes positively charged in comparison with the outside of the cell.

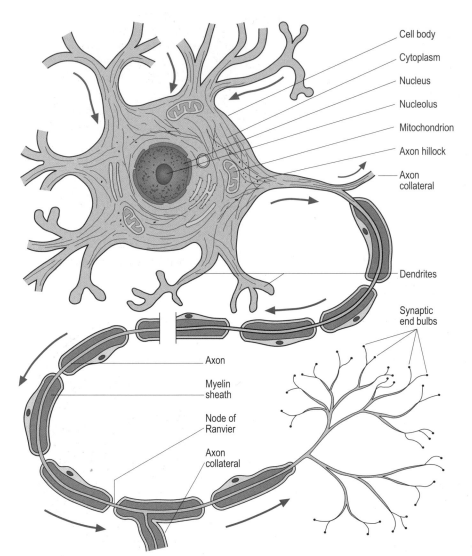

Cell body
Cytoplasm
Nucleus
Nucleolus
Mitochondrion
Axon hillock
Axon collateral
Dendrites
Synaptic end bulbs
Axon
Myelin sheath
Node of Ranvier
Axon collateral

Figure 8.2 Anatomy of a typical neuron.

The next region of the axon will still be maintaining its resting potential and because unlike charges attract, the positive ions within the cell will be attracted towards the area of negativity; thus the impulse will spread down the length of the axon.

Once a section of the cell membrane has become depolarized, K^+ ions leak out of the cells and the sodium channels close again, so restoring the resting potential. This is called repolarization. Until resting potential has been restored, the neuron cannot respond to another stimulus.

The whole cycle from resting potential, through depolarization and repolarization and back to resting potential, takes only a millisecond and when stimulated, up to 200 action potentials/s can be passed along the neuron.

Transmission of information

An action potential occurs as the result of stimulation of a dendrite by a stimulus. This stimulus may be the result of a sensation that needs to be

(a)

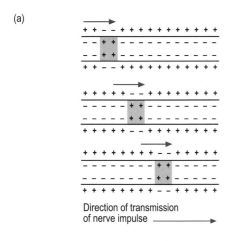

Direction of transmission
of nerve impulse

(b)

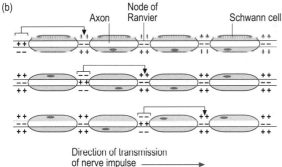

Direction of transmission
of nerve impulse

Figure 8.3 Conduction of an impulse in a neuron.
(a) Unmyelinated neuron. (b) Myelinated neuron.

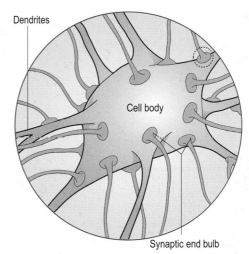

Figure 8.4 Relationship between synaptic end bulbs
and cell bodies

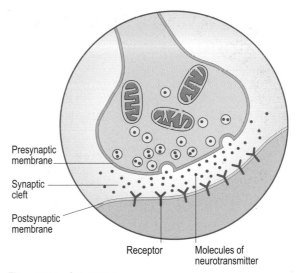

Figure 8.5 A synapse.

sent to the cerebral cortex or may be in response to the interpretation of sensory input requiring an action or a motor output such as contraction of a muscle. Senses that stimulate an action impulse can take many forms. These may be touch, light, heat or damage to organs or tissues, changes in ion concentration, chemical concentration, or pressure. As a result of dendritic stimulation, an action potential is triggered in the neuron detecting the sensation. However, this neuron does not stretch all the way from the source of the stimulus to the brain. Several neurons are found along the pathway. Thus, the stimulus must be passed from one neuron to the next. At the terminal end of the neuron, branches of the axon extend in several potential directions ending with a synaptic end bulb. Synapses are present between synaptic end bulbs and dendrites of the adjoining neurons. Dendrites and cell bodies are often covered in synaptic end bulbs from many different neurons (Fig. 8.4).

A synapse is a space across which an action potential must be transmitted. This process is carried out by the production of a chemical by the terminal synaptic end bulb. This substance diffuses across the space and results in an increase or decrease in the permeability of the cell wall of the dendrite of the adjoining neuron (Fig. 8.5). Thus, an action potential will be initiated or the impulse inhibited from spreading along the axon of the receiving neuron. In this capacity, these chemicals are known as neurotransmitters.

Neurotransmitters are synthesized in the synaptic end bulb or in the cell body of the neuron; in the latter case the chemical will need to be transported along the axon to the synapse. Many chemicals perform this function including acetylcholine and dopamine, oxytocin and the endorphins.

EPILEPSY

Epilepsy is a condition in which abnormal electrical activity in the brain generates inappropriate action potentials resulting in strange sensations, behaviour, muscle spasm or seizures. Most people will be familiar with the sight of an individual having a typical spasmodic fit. However, there are several types of epilepsy and these are described below.

Aetiology

In the normal brain, there is a balance between excitation and inhibition within and between neurons. In some forms of epilepsy, this balance is lost and neurons in a small region or over an extensive area have an increased level of excitation. Action potentials are triggered spontaneously in these regions and spread in a haphazard manner. Abnormal electrical activity may remain within a small area of the brain or spread over large areas of the brain. The cause of an increase in excitation is commonly unknown and this form of epilepsy is classified as idiopathic.

Other causes include:

- Physical causes, such as head injury, cerebral tumours, stroke, hypertension, infection
- Congenital defects, such as cerebral palsy, intracranial cysts
- Metabolic causes, such as hyperglycaemia, hypoxia, uraemia, fluid and electrolyte imbalance, hypernatraemia, alcohol, drugs
- Syndromes, such as Alzheimer's, Wernicke–Korsakoff, Wilson's disease (Lavan 2006).

There is some evidence that there is a genetic component which predisposes some individuals to epileptic seizures.

Incidence

Epilepsy is one of the most common of the neurological disorders. It affects people of all ages, irrespective of geographical location, gender or race. The incidence of epilepsy in developed countries is around 50/100 000 per year and is higher in children and the elderly (MacDonald et al 2000). The occurrence of epilepsy in childhood in developed countries has fallen over the past three decades and is thought to be due to the improved health of pregnant women, regular prenatal care and the availability of immunization programmes (Duncan et al 2006). It is thought that about one person in 20 has a seizure at one time in their lives but these may not be due to epilepsy (www.epilepsy.org.uk). The incidence of epilepsy is approximately 1 in 150 people (NICE 2004). Epilepsy of unknown cause occurs most commonly in the under 20s.

Signs and symptoms

Epilepsy is not a distinct disease but a group of disorders in which recurrent seizures are the main symptom. Seizures occur as a result of an underlying pathological process in the brain and can thus take many forms. Some seizures also appear to be triggered by an external factor. Stress, alcohol, heat and exhaustion have all been implicated in stimulating seizures, as has exposure to strobe lighting. The majority of seizures however, occur spontaneously.

Seizures are described according to whether their onset is focal or generalized. Focal or partial seizures may be classified as being a simple seizure in which consciousness is retained throughout or a complex seizure if consciousness is impaired at some point.

Simple partial seizure

This type of seizure occurs when a small area of the brain is disturbed by a stimulus resulting in disruption of function of that part of the brain. Often this occurs in a small part of the motor cortex. The patient experiences a twitching of the muscles of the side of the face or typically the thumb but does not lose consciousness. Rarely, this spreads to other adjacent areas of the body and is then described as a Jacksonian seizure (Walsh 2002).

Complex partial seizure

A complex partial seizure often originates in the temporal lobe and is usually preceded by an aura or warning. The patient then demonstrates a series of repeated movements, such as rubbing of the hands or plucking at clothes. This is described as automatism. The patient may also experience an abnormal sensory sensation such as a smell or a sense of *déjà vu*.

Generalized seizures (tonic clonic seizures)

These seizures are those commonly recognized as the typical 'grand mal' epileptic fit. Several distinct stages occur:

- Aura: This may be experienced as a strange taste in the mouth or other inappropriate sensation. Not all patients experience an identifiable aura. Once recognized by the patient, the aura enables her to alert others and move to a safe place

- Loss of consciousness: The patient will lose consciousness. She will fall to the ground if standing and therefore may injure herself

- Tonic stage: During this stage, there is generalized contraction of the muscles of the body. The patient may be incontinent as the muscles of the bladder and bowel contract and she may utter a cry as the air is forcibly ejected from the lungs. Respiratory muscles also contract and ventilation ceases resulting in gradually increasing cyanosis

- Clonic stage: Muscles now undergo rhythmic contraction and relaxation. Limbs jerk violently and there is frothing at the mouth from the overproduction of saliva

- Coma: Finally, all movement ceases and the patient falls into a coma. Breathing returns to normal and cyanosis disappears. On waking, often several hours later, the patient is confused, partially amnesic and drowsy.

Not all generalized seizures go through all these stages. Tonic seizures may occur where the patient suddenly loses body posture and both arms and legs flex for a brief period of time. The patient loses consciousness and becomes cyanosed. Tonic atonic seizures may also be experienced where the tonic seizure described above is followed by a period of complete loss of muscular tone, often repeated several times. Again, there is loss of consciousness.

Other variations in types of seizures are ones in which the patient loses awareness for a few seconds – an absence, commonly called a 'petit mal' seizure, sometimes accompanied by a period of automatism, or myoclonic seizures in which one or more limbs jerk repeatedly over a number of hours. Brief periods of loss of consciousness may occur.

Status epilepticus

The occasional epileptic seizure may occur in any patient if they are unwell or their medication does not control the condition. However, this should be an isolated single seizure. A serious complication of epilepsy is the occurrence of status epilepticus in which the patient has repeated generalized seizures with no recovery of normal alertness between them. The patient develops hyperpyrexia, a deepening coma and will suffer brain damage due to the continuing cyanosis. If not rapidly treated, the patient will become completely exhausted, severely hypoxic and death may occur. Treatment is with intravenous lorazepam 4 mg or diazepam 10 mg (Hayes 2004). Status epilepticus is associated with abrupt discontinuation of anticonvulsant medication or inadequately treated epilepsy.

Diagnosis

Having one seizure does not indicate that a person has epilepsy. In infancy, seizures are a relatively common complication of acute infection associated with high temperature – a febrile convulsion. Experiencing one or more seizures in pregnancy as a complication of a hypertensive disorder rarely leads to further seizures once treated and the pregnancy terminated (see Ch. 2).

Epilepsy is suspected if a patient has two or more seizures not related to a systemic disorder such as those described above. The patient should be urgently referred to an epilepsy specialist who can get the condition under control as quickly as possible (NICE 2004). Diagnosis is based on an accurate clinical observation of the occurrence and pattern of seizures from a reliable witness. A complete physical and neurological examination would then be carried out. Blood samples would be sent for laboratory examination to rule out a metabolic cause. Diagnosis can then be confirmed by further investigations as necessary, such as lumbar puncture, electroencephalogram (EEG) and magnetic resonance investigation (MRI).

Treatment

Once epilepsy is diagnosed, it is important to begin treatment as soon as possible. For over 60% of those diagnosed with epilepsy, seizures can be controlled with modern medicines and surgical techniques (Sander 2003).

Antiepileptic drugs are the mainstay of treatment (Box 8.1). Non-pharmacological treatments are normally only considered when antiepileptic medications have been tried and have not been successful in preventing seizures. Surgery may be required and some success has been achieved using the ketogenic diet in children.

Box 8.1 Med alert tags

A medical identification tag is a small tag worn as a bracelet, necklace or on clothing, identifying that the wearer has a serious medical condition which may affect the way they are to be treated. The intention of this tag is to alert health professionals or emergency services that the wearer has the condition, when she is not conscious enough to explain. The tag carries a reference number enabling the health professional to access information about the wearer's medical condition and treatment. Some people prefer to carry a card in their wallet with the same information. The latest technology provides a USB device that is identifiable as a med alert tag. The wearer can update the information regularly and the information is readily available through any computer system.

A wide range of effective antiepileptic drugs are available to treat the different forms of epilepsy. The neurologist will select suitable medication based on the patient's age and weight, and the type, frequency and cause of the seizures. The dosage is gradually built up over several months until seizures are controlled in order to reduce adverse reactions. An alternative or additional medication should not be used until the maximum dose of the previous drug has been reached.

There are three mechanisms by which antiepileptic drugs exert their effects (Jordan 2002):

1. By limiting the sustained repetitive firing of neurons by altering the ability of the nerve cell membranes to transport ions such as sodium – carbamazepine, phenytoin, sodium valproate.
2. By effecting inhibition at the synapse – gabapentin, vigabatrin.
3. By acting on calcium ion channels in the thalamus – ethosuximide, sodium valproate.

The mechanism of action of these drugs is not fully understood and many have multiple effects (Duncan et al 2006). Most of these drugs have side-effects, especially when first prescribed – symptoms such as drowsiness, nausea or skin irritation. The aim of treatment is to find a single drug which controls the seizures at the lowest effective dose with the minimum of side-effects.

There are some individuals who do not respond to a single drug and polytherapy is necessary. The use of several drugs increases the chance of non-compliance, drug interaction and long-term side-effects (Duncan et al 2006).

In some patients, seizures cannot be controlled by antiepileptic medication. Surgery is the only option. A localized area of damaged tissue is removed from the relevant part of the brain. This is not without risks and complications, such as memory loss, and language difficulties have been reported in patients who have had left-temporal lobe surgery (www.epilepsy.org.uk). Another alternative is to have a vagal nerve stimulator inserted to abort seizures. This can however cause adverse reactions, such as dyspnoea, hoarseness, cough and tingling in the neck.

A point to note for women of childbearing age is that some antiepileptic drugs can interfere with the effectiveness of oral contraceptives (Doggett-Jones 2007). Also the physician caring for a woman of childbearing age should consider the teratogenic effect of the drugs being considered and try to stabilize her epileptic condition on drugs with the least risk of congenital defects should the woman subsequently become pregnant.

Education of the patient is a vital part of the treatment process. Empowering the patient to observe signs and symptoms that may precede a seizure will inform the neurologist and enable the patient to take appropriate action. It is essential to teach the patient to avoid known seizure triggers, such as fatigue, fever, caffeine, stress, excess alcohol and flickering lights (Lavan 2006). Encouraging a healthy lifestyle with a well balanced diet, exercise and sufficient sleep will minimize the number of seizures experienced (Lanfear 2002).

Prognosis

Most people with epilepsy lead outwardly normal lives. While epilepsy cannot currently be cured, treatment of an underlying disease process may stop the seizures occurring. However, often the cause is not known or it is not possible to treat the cause. Despite the existence of many different antiepileptic drugs, one-third of individuals with epilepsy continue to suffer seizures (Kwan & Sander 2004). In these cases, epilepsy and the seizures that result do not progress to cause brain damage unless status epilepticus occurs.

It is not uncommon however for people with epilepsy, especially children, to develop behavioural and emotional problems, sometimes as a result of embarrassment and frustration or bullying and teasing with subsequent avoidance of school and other social settings (Freeman et al 2003). Epilepsy is associated with a wide range of markers of social and economic disadvantage, such as poor academic achievement, low income or unemployment.

For many people with epilepsy, the risk of seizures may restrict their independence. Driving is banned unless the individual has been free of seizures for 1 year, or free from seizures during the day. The DVLA also recommends that patients who are having their medication withdrawn should not drive until 6 months after the medication has been discontinued.

Rarely, an individual with epilepsy may die unexpectedly. Sudden unexplained death in epilepsy (SUDEP) is uncommon but is a recognized syndrome where a person with epilepsy dies suddenly and no other cause of death is found (www.SUDEP.org). Sudden unexplained deaths happen in people without epilepsy but individuals with epilepsy appear to have an increased risk. SUDEP has been shown to be related to seizures but the severity and frequency of the seizures does not appear to be implicated in the incidence of this condition. Risks are however negligible in those who are seizure free. Overall, the risk of SUDEP is 1 in 1000 cases/year, which accounts for 500 deaths/year in the UK (Hanna et al 2002).

Other causes of premature death in individuals with epilepsy include trauma, suicide, pneumonia and status epilepticus (Gaitatzis & Sander 2004). It is thought that symptomatic epilepsy can reduce life expectancy by 18 years (Gaitatzis et al 2004).

EPILEPSY IN PREGNANCY

Caring for a woman with epilepsy requires a multidisciplinary team approach. As the primary care giver in the majority of pregnancies including those of high risk, it is vital that the midwife has a good understanding of the condition, of its treatment and its effect on the woman and her fetus/neonate.

Pregnancy brings considerable changes to the physiology of the body, which may affect a woman with epilepsy. Therapeutic levels of antiepileptic drugs may be disrupted by circulatory changes or by nausea and vomiting. Psychological stress is also increased in pregnancy and this may contribute to the increased risk of seizures. The hormones of pregnancy can affect the seizure threshold (Jordan 2002).

Women with epilepsy who plan to become pregnant therefore face a difficult decision: to continue treatment with antiepileptic medication and accept the increased risk for birth defects or to stop medication and accept the risk of uncontrolled seizures, which may compromise their own health and are potentially harmful to the fetus. The management of women with epilepsy during pregnancy therefore presents a major clinical dilemma (Kälviäinen & Tomson 2006).

In some women, consideration may be given to reduce or cease medication, as this is the best option for them and their fetus (Lewis & Drife 2004). This does however increase the risk of seizures and in the Confidential Enquiries into Maternal deaths 2000–2002, there were 13 deaths from epilepsy. The majority of these were probably due to SUDEP, which is likely in those having seizures. Aspiration was another major contributing factor. Two women died however as a result of having had their antiepileptic medication reduced or ceased altogether because of concern over the effect it might have on the fetus.

Physiological changes in pregnancy

During pregnancy, there are considerable changes to body systems. In the cardiovascular system, there is an increase in plasma volume of 50% with a corresponding increase in blood cells and proteins of about 20% to meet the increasing demands of both the mother and her fetus. This will result in a dilution in circulating volume of any drugs that are being transported in the bloodstream, either dissolved in plasma or attached to proteins. This may result in drug levels dropping beneath the therapeutic level that is required to control epileptic seizures (Box 8.2). If the pregnancy is then complicated by excessive fluid retention caused by, for example, one of the hypertensive disorders of pregnancy, this will aggravate the difficulty in maintaining therapeutic levels of the antiepileptic drugs in the bloodstream.

Oestrogen and progesterone also have an effect on epilepsy. Oestrogen increases activity of the foci that trigger seizures, while progesterone dampens their activity (Blackburn 2002). As pregnancy progresses, the levels of these hormones alter and affect the threshold at which seizures may occur. Sodium and water retention may aggravate this, as may the mild respiratory alkalosis of pregnancy.

Box 8.2 Pharmacokinetics

Pharmacokinetics describes how the body handles a drug. It describes absorption, distribution and elimination. Every drug has a therapeutic range – that is a top limit above which toxic effects may appear and a bottom limit below which the drug will not have the desired effect. For some drugs, the therapeutic range is very narrow and some antiepileptic drugs are in this category. These drugs may need regular measurements of plasma concentration.

The concentration of a drug within the body depends on the way the drug is handled by the body. Most drugs are taken orally because this is most convenient. Generally, drugs are absorbed through the walls of the small intestine. In pregnancy, there is a delay in this process due to the decrease in gut mobility under the influence of progesterone. This may reduce the efficacy of the drugs.

Distribution of drugs is usually affected by the availability of plasma proteins to which they bind for transportation and the degree to which they are lipid soluble. In pregnancy, the number of plasma proteins may be reduced, particularly if there is renal damage. This may increase the effect and side-effects of some drugs. Distribution is also dependent on an adequate circulation.

The route of elimination varies with individual drugs. Some require metabolizing before they can be excreted from the body. Others are removed largely unaltered. Dysfunction of the renal and/or hepatic system may prevent normal elimination of the drugs and a build up of the drug above the therapeutic range.

Incidence

In many women with epilepsy, pregnancy is unplanned due to the increased risk of contraceptive failure of 7/100 women years. 1 in 250 pregnant women suffer from epilepsy (SIGN 2003).

Preconception advice

All women should be offered preconception advice by a member of the multidisciplinary team, whether they suffer from a condition such as epilepsy or not. The woman with epilepsy should however receive careful advice and management regarding the drug medication that she has been using to control her epileptic seizures. Women who are regularly seen by a practice nurse are more likely to receive preconception advice (Hayes 2004).

All antiepileptic medication has an effect on the developing fetus and therefore the woman's drugs should be carefully reviewed. Neural tube defects occur in 1–2% of pregnancies in woman with epilepsy who are treated with sodium valproate or carbamazepine (Genton & Gelisse 2002). However, women on antiepileptic drugs develop folic acid deficiency and this may be a factor in this incidence. Phenytoin has been shown to increase the risk to the developing embryo of craniofacial malformations and growth retardation (Lloyd 2003). Establishing the woman on one of the safer drugs well before pregnancy is contemplated will greatly reduce the risks of teratogenesis (Tennenborn 2006). Polytherapy is associated with a significantly increased risk of congenital abnormality (Morrow et al 2005). Folic acid supplementation of 5 mg/day should also be commenced before pregnancy and continued throughout pregnancy.

Pregnancy

Care for the woman with epilepsy should be provided by a multidisciplinary team, preferably at a combined clinic to prevent multiple hospital appointments. A midwife should always be present at the clinic to ensure that the woman and her family have the opportunity to discuss any aspect of her pregnancy with the health professional that will be providing the majority of her care.

Women with epilepsy have a higher rate of complications in pregnancy than generally. The aetiology of these complications is unclear, however (Fitzgerald 2004). It is uncertain whether the complications associated with epilepsy are due to the genetics of the condition, the seizures or the use of antiepileptic medication. Reported complications include fetal abnormalities, spontaneous abortion, stillbirth, placental defects, placental abruption, pre-term labour, hypertensive disorders and haemorrhage (Foldvary 2001).

Epilepsy in pregnancy is usefully discussed by considering the effect of epilepsy on pregnancy and that of the pregnancy on the condition and its treatment.

Effect of epilepsy on pregnancy

Many women with epilepsy suffer from sub-fertility (Hamed et al 2006).

As discussed above, many antiepileptic drugs are thought to damage the fetus if taken early in pregnancy. It is therefore essential that a woman with epilepsy should have her pregnancy monitored very carefully to identify any consequences of this medication. Maternal serum alpha-fetoprotein will be offered at 15–20 weeks' gestation and an early anomaly scan at 18–20 weeks, to rule out fetal abnormalities. The woman should be thoroughly advised of the risks to her baby of non-compliance with medication – the danger to the fetus of the woman having seizures is greater than the risk from the medications.

As well as folic acid, it is important that the woman is advised to commence vitamin D supplementation as antiepileptic drugs are known to disrupt absorption of this vital nutrient.

Effect of pregnancy on the condition

Most women who have their epilepsy well controlled before pregnancy commences, have a trouble free pregnancy. However, some women experience an increase in seizures. Approximately 40% of women will demonstrate an increase in seizure frequency; 8% a decrease in frequency; and around 50% will stay the same (Blackburn 2002). Seizures may reappear after many seizure-free years or may occur for the first time in pregnancy. Most women return to their pre-pregnancy pattern postnatally.

One of the possible causes of this change in seizure pattern may be the circulatory changes described above. Circulatory changes will affect the maintenance of therapeutic levels of drugs in the bloodstream. (Box 8.2). Therapeutic drug levels will therefore be monitored on a regular basis and dosage adjusted accordingly (Adab et al 2001).

Therapeutic levels will be further disrupted if absorption of the drugs is prevented by the woman suffering from nausea and vomiting in early pregnancy.

Labour

Labour is a time of increased stress and lack of sleep, overbreathing, pain and dehydration – all factors that may trigger an epileptic seizure. Seizures are more common in labour with 2–3% of all labouring women having a grand mal seizure (Greenhill & Betts 2003). Care of the woman with epilepsy should therefore be the same as all other women, maintaining as normal a birthing process as is possible. Antiepileptic medication should be continued throughout labour and the midwife should be vigilant for signs of an impending seizure.

The puerperium

Postnatally, the risks associated with epilepsy are related to caring for the baby. The mother should be advised how to minimize risk when feeding, bathing, changing and transporting her baby. Breast-feeding is encouraged as antiepileptic drugs are present in very low levels in breast milk. Caring for a young baby is however associated with fatigue and sleep deprivation and the mother should be encouraged to take up offers of support wherever possible.

Antiepileptic medication should be reviewed after 6 weeks, with a view to returning dosage to pre-pregnancy levels. Contraceptive advice will be given and the mother advised to attend for preconception advice before embarking on another pregnancy. The mother should be advised about the risk of failure of the contraceptive pill with some of the antiepileptic medications (Harden 2006) but there is no method of contraception that is not suitable for the women with epilepsy.

The midwife's management of the pregnant woman with epilepsy

The role of the midwife as in any pregnancy complicated by a medical condition is to support the woman and her family and ensure that the pregnancy is treated as normal as far as is possible. Pregnancies complicated in this way are considered high risk and as such, are much more likely to become 'managed'. The midwife's role is to include the woman and her family in all the decisions made so that the woman can make her own informed choices in care. As in all complicated pregnancies, there are many opportunities to encourage good outcome by giving the woman the options and advice that encourage physiological birth.

Most women with epilepsy will have received preconception advice on the effect their condition will have on their pregnancy and their newborn baby. However, the midwife must have a good working knowledge of the condition in order to clarify and educate the woman on the condition itself and the effect her antiepileptic medication will have on her pregnancy and, usually of great concern to the woman, on the health of her unborn child.

Before pregnancy or as early in pregnancy as possible, the midwife should discuss with the woman her family, medical and obstetric history. This 'booking visit' can be considered as an opportunity to do a risk assessment of the pregnancy in order to identify areas of potential concern. Having taken a careful history of her epilepsy, the midwife is then in a position to advise her appropriately. This pregnancy will be supervised by the multidisciplinary team, as the presence of epilepsy removes the pregnancy from the midwife's normal sphere of practice (NMC 2004).

Pregnancy

At each visit to the multidisciplinary team, the woman should have an opportunity to see her midwife. The midwife should advise the woman on her own safety throughout pregnancy should a seizure occur, and postnatally of how to safely care for her baby.

In pregnancy, issues such as bathing when there is someone in the house are advised as is the danger of stimulating a seizure if the bath water is too warm. This latter point should be raised with all pregnant women as they are at increased risk of fainting due to the drop in blood pressure during the second trimester of pregnancy.

Management of a seizure

A generalized epileptic seizure is an emergency which occurs usually without warning but is over very quickly. The priorities in management for the midwife are to prevent the patient from injuring herself and to observe the sequence of events for discussion with the medical practitioners.

During the seizure, the midwife must stay with the woman and monitor her condition but send for medical aid if possible. The midwife should remain calm and reassure those in attendance. No attempt must be made to restrain the patient during the fit or to insert any instrument into the mouth in the mistaken belief that this will prevent the patient from biting her tongue. However, it is essential to prevent the woman from damaging herself and therefore the midwife must remove any objects in the vicinity that could cause injury. Pillows can be removed to lay the woman flat or if she has collapsed to the floor cover her with a blanket, insert a pillow under her head to prevent injury and observe until the seizure ceases. If available, oxygen can be administered by placing the mask close to her face. Due to the risks from aspiration, it would be useful to roll her onto her side if this does not limit her movement during the seizure.

During a seizure, the midwife should make the following observations:

- Did there appear to be an aura?
- In which part of the body did the seizure commence?
- Were the movements localized or generalized and if the latter, were these symmetrical?
- Did the woman become cyanosed?
- Was there clenching of the teeth or frothing at the mouth?
- Was there incontinence of urine or faeces?
- How long did each stage of the seizure last?

Once the seizure has ceased, the woman should be made comfortable in bed in the recovery position, to avoid any risk of aspiration, and her vitals should be noted. A cardiotocograph should be completed if appropriate. She should remain under close observation with cot sides raised until she has fully recovered, as she may be disorientated when she first recovers consciousness.

If this seizure is followed quickly by another, this may be status epilepticus. This is a medical emergency and medical aid must be obtained as quickly as possible. The woman will quickly become exhausted and hypoxic and this may have a devastating effect on both the mother and the fetus.

The neonate

A total of 4–8% of babies born to women with epilepsy who are on antiepileptic medication will have a congenital anomaly. This is 2–3 times higher than in the general population (Pennell 2003). Phenytoin is one of the most commonly prescribed antiepileptic medications and has been associated with fetal hydantoin syndrome, which consists of intrauterine growth restriction, with facial clefts and heart defects (Barrett & Richens 2003). However, many of the antiepileptic medications have the potential to harm the fetus.

Vitamin K levels are lower than normal in the fetus of a woman with epilepsy – antiepileptic medication crosses the placenta and speeds up vitamin K metabolism (Pennell 2003). This vitamin must therefore be administered to the fetus immediately after delivery to prevent haemorrhagic disease of the newborn. Administration of vitamin K to the mother from the 36th week of pregnancy may prevent this (Kaaja et al 2002).

The behaviour of the neonate may also be affected by the presence of the drugs in the bloodstream until they are totally excreted from his body. Many of these infants will be reluctant feeders and gain weight slowly. A minority of babies will show withdrawal symptoms, such as irritability or convulsions.

Future pregnancies

During the postnatal period, the midwife is in an ideal position to educate the woman about the effects of epilepsy on fertility and future pregnancies. Crawford & Hudson (2003) found that over one-third of actual or potential users of the oral contraceptive pill had not been told about its potential interaction with antiepileptic drugs. Additionally, the majority of women asked were not aware that there was an increased risk of congenital abnormality with antiepileptic drugs if taken at conception. The midwife will be able to advise women to take advice before conception on the drugs she is taking to control seizures. Crawford & Hudson (2003) also found that one-third of the women studied had voluntarily decided not to have children because of the risks involved.

MULTIPLE SCLEROSIS

Around 85 000 people in the UK suffer from multiple sclerosis (MS). MS is a disorder in which the myelin sheath that surrounds the nerve cells of the nervous system is progressively destroyed and replaced with scar tissue in the form of hardened white plaques or sclera. The axons themselves become affected by the process and degenerate gradually over time. MS is thought to occur secondary to an autoimmune response.

As discussed above, the myelin sheath acts as 'lagging' on the axon of the neuron preventing loss of ions between the cell and the surrounding fluid. The result of the presence of myelin is to enable an action potential to move extremely rapidly along the neuron – much faster than neurons without myelin. Loss of myelin will therefore interrupt or slow down the functioning of that particular nerve pathway. In MS, signs and symptoms and the severity of the condition depend on where the myelin has been destroyed and to what extent the underlying axon has degenerated.

Multiple sclerosis affects 40–60 people per 100 000 population worldwide but there is a marked geographical variance. People in cold damp climates are particularly vulnerable and in Scotland, the incidence rises to 100–300 per 100 000 (Walsh 2002). The disease tends to appear in the under 30s and there is a slightly higher incidence in women.

The effect on the patient varies widely from one patient to another according to which part of the nervous system is affected. The optic and cervical spinal cord tends to be afflicted initially in many people. MS is characterized by relapses and remissions and the process of the disease is largely unpredictable. Prognosis varies from an initial onset of symptoms which then go into permanent remission, to a malignant aggressive degeneration

in which there is no remission and death occurs within a few weeks. More commonly, patients with MS lead relatively normal lives for many years after its onset before becoming increasingly debilitated after each relapse. Most patients survive more than 20 years after the initial onset.

Onset of the disease commonly develops after a stressful experience such as anxiety, trauma, infection or pregnancy. Signs and symptoms vary considerably between patients dependent on the sites of damage. These may include extreme fatigue, visual dysfunction, numbness, tingling or loss of sensation, muscular weakness or personality changes. Some return to normal functioning may occur but deficits that persist beyond 3 months are unlikely to recover.

There is no cure for MS and treatment can only be symptomatic and supportive. Physiotherapy encourages mobility and independence. Corticosteroids are used during severe relapses.

Pregnancy does not seem to affect the course of the disease, nor does MS affect pregnancy outcome. Provided disability is not so severe as to limit ability to perform parenting tasks, there is no real reason to limit the number of pregnancies. However, the woman with MS will need a great deal of support during pregnancy and subsequently with childcare.

MYASTHENIA GRAVIS

Clinical manifestations of this condition include variable weakness and fatigue of skeletal muscles caused by defective neuromuscular transmission. The disorder is probably the result of an autoimmune response and is characterized by a reduced number of acetylcholine receptors at the neuromuscular junction. It is more common in women than in men and may appear for the first time in pregnancy or shortly afterwards. The effect of the disease on pregnancy varies and is unpredictable. The effects on the neonate may mimic the disease on the mother but these effects are usually transient and do not predict disease in the adult. Termination of pregnancy does not appear to benefit those with worsening disease during pregnancy. In fact, the postpartum period may be the most dangerous time regardless of the length of pregnancy. If pre-term labour occurs, the use of magnesium sulphate is absolutely contraindicated as it interferes with the already defective neuromuscular transmission by altering the exchange of ions across the synapse (Blackburn 2002).

Myasthenia gravis is a relatively rare condition but one in which the incidence is at its highest between the ages of 20 and 30 years. Women are affected more often than men. Around 15/100 000 of the population are affected at any one time, although it is thought that the condition is underdiagnosed.

Myasthenia gravis presents as a weakness of the muscles that control eye and eyelid movements, facial expression, chewing, talking and swallowing. The patient complains that the severity of the weakness progresses during the day, improving after periods of rest. Weakness is restricted to the ocular muscles in many patients.

Treatment options include the use of immunosuppressants. Surgery is also an option – removal of the thymus gland improves or in some cases cures the patient. The prognosis for the patient with myasthenia gravis is usually quite good. She can expect to lead a normal or near normal life. Remission occurs in some cases. Pregnancy however, is one of the conditions that can cause worsening of this condition. Other factors that can negatively affect the course of this disease are disorders of the thyroid, respiratory infections and emotional upset.

CEREBROVASCULAR ACCIDENT (STROKE)

A cerebrovascular accident (CVA) also known as a stroke is an acute neurological injury in which the blood supply to a part of the brain is interrupted. Lack of blood results in lack of oxygen and nutrients to that part of the brain and subsequent death of the cells. Functioning of that part of the brain is lost. CVA is a leading cause of death in those over 60 years of age but can occur in younger people and thus a midwife needs to be aware of the possibility of this occurring in the women for whom she cares.

The commonest cause of a CVA is partial occlusion of a blood vessel due to the build up of a thrombus around plaques of atherosclerosis.

This results in ischaemia of the tissues supplied by that artery and resulting dysfunction of that area of the brain. Another possible cause is blockage of a blood vessel by an embolism which has been produced elsewhere in the body and travels to the brain where it lodges in the small blood vessels (see Ch. 4). Haemorrhage is another possible cause – this may be due to a weakness in the blood vessel or the presence of an aneurysm. The resulting rupture of the blood vessel damages the neural tissue, either from pressure due to the presence of the clot, or by cell death as a consequence of lack of blood to the area supplied by that blood vessel.

The symptoms of a stroke depend on the area in which the CVA has occurred. Examples of these are:

- Speech defects or inability to make voluntary movements will be due to a defect in the cerebral cortex

- Muscle weakness or diminished sensory perception will be the result of damage to one of the principal nerve pathways through the brain

- Uncoordinated movements or difficulty in walking may suggest the stroke has occurred in the cerebellum.

Treatment of the CVA depends both on its cause and on its location. Clot busting drugs can be used if the cause is a thrombus or embolism. Surgery may be required if the stroke has been caused by haemorrhage. Whatever the cause and the success of the treatment, the mainstay of future care is rehabilitation, which involves re-learning the functions that have been lost.

Some 95% of cerebrovascular accidents occur in those over the age of 45. However, this condition can occur at any age including in a fetus. Some families seem to have an increased tendency to suffer stroke. Women have increased risk factors, such as pregnancy, the use of oral contraceptives, the menopause and the use of hormone replacement therapy.

The risk of suffering a stroke can be reduced dramatically by modifying a person's lifestyle. Smoking cessation, a healthier diet, reducing alcohol intake and screening for high cholesterol levels can all reduce the risks considerably.

REFERENCES

Adab N, Jacoby A, Smith D, Chadwick D 2001 Additional educational needs in children born to mothers with epilepsy. Journal of Neurology Neurosurgery and Psychiatry 70:15–21

Barrett C, Richens A 2003 Epilepsy and pregnancy: Report of an epilepsy research foundation workshop. Epilepsy Research 52:147–187

Blackburn S 2002 Maternal, fetal and neonatal physiology: A clinical perspective, 2nd edn. WB Saunders, Philadelphia, p 255–309

Crawford P, Hudson S 2003 Understanding the information needs of women with epilepsy at different life stages. Seizure 12(7):502–507

Doggett-Jones S 2007 Contraception for women with epilepsy. Practise Nurse 33(4):32–37

Duncan J S, Sander J W, Sisodiya S M, Walker M C 2006 Adult epilepsy. Lancet 367:1087–1100

Fitzgerald K E 2004 Use of phenytoin in pregnancy for epileptic seizure prevention: a case report. Journal of Midwifery & Women's Health 49(2):145–147

Foldvary N 2001 Treatment issues for women with epilepsy. Clinical Neurology 19:409–425

Freeman J M, Vining E P G, Pillas D J 2003 Seizures and epilepsy in childhood: A guide for parents, 3rd edn. John Hopkins University Press, Baltimore

Gaitatzis A, Sander J W 2004 The mortality of epilepsy revisited. Epileptic Disorders 6:3–13

Gaitatzis A, Johnson A L, Chadwick D W et al 2004 Life expectancy in people with *newly* diagnosed epilepsy. Brain 127:2427–2432

Genton P, Gelisse P 2002 Valproate acid. Adverse effects. In: Levy R, Mattson R, Meldrum B, Perruca E (eds) Antiepileptic drugs, 5th edn. Lippincott, Williams and Wilkins, London, p 844–845

Greenhill L, Betts T 2003 The lifelong needs of women with epilepsy. Practice Nursing 14(7):302–309

Hamed S A, Hamed E A, Shokry M, Omar H, Abdellah M M 2006 Reproductive conditions and lipid profiles in females with epilepsy. Drugs 66(14):1817–1829

Hanna J, Black M, Sander J W et al 2002 Death in the shadows: the national sentinel clinical audit into epilepsy death. National Institute for Clinical Excellence (NICE), London

Harden C L 2006 Optimising therapy of seizures in women who use oral contraceptives. Neurology 67(12):S56–S58

Hayes C 2004 Clinical skills: practical guide for managing adults with epilepsy. British Journal of Nursing 13(7):380–387

Jordan S 2002 Pharmacology for midwives. Palgrave, Houndmills

Kaaja E, Kaaja R, Matila R, Hiilesmaa V 2002 Enzyme inducing antiepileptic drugs in pregnancy: The risk of bleeding in the neonate. Neurology 58:549–553

Kälviäinen R, Tomson T 2006 Optimising treatment of epilepsy during pregnancy. Neurology 67(12):S59–S63

Kwan P, Sander J W 2004 The natural history of epilepsy: An epidemiological view. Journal of Neurology Neurosurgery and Psychiatry 75:1376–1381

Lanfear J 2002 The individual with epilepsy. Nursing Standard 16(46):43–55

Lavan Z P 2006 Epilepsy: Out of the shadows. Journal of Community Nursing 20(9):4–12

Lewis G, Drife J eds 2004 Why Mothers Die 2000–2002: The sixth report of the Confidential Enquires into Maternal Deaths in the United Kingdom. RCOG, London

Lloyd C 2003 Common medical disorders associated with pregnancy. In: Fraser DM, Cooper MA (eds) Myles textbook for midwives. Churchill Livingstone, Edinburgh, p 321–355

MacDonald B K, Cockerell O C, Sander J W et al 2000. The incidence and lifetime prevalence of neurological disorders in a prospective community-based study in the UK. Brain 123:665–676

Morrow J M, Russell A, Guthrie E et al 2005 Malformation risks of antiepileptic drugs in pregnancy: A prospective study from the UK Epilepsy and Pregnancy Register. Journal of Neurology Neurosurgery and Psychiatry 77(2):193–198

National Institute for Clinical Excellence 2004 The epilepsies: the diagnosis and management of epilepsies in adults and children in primary and secondary care. Guideline 20. NICE, London

Nursing and Midwifery Council (NMC) 2004 Midwives rules and standards. NMC, London

Pennell P 2003 Antiepileptic drug pharmacokinetics during pregnancy and lactation. Neurology 61:S35–42

Sander J W 2003 The epidemiology of epilepsy revisited. Current Opinion in Neurology 16:165–170

Scottish Intercollegiate Guidelines Network 2003 Diagnosis and management of epilepsy in adults. SIGN, Edinburgh

Tennenborn B 2006 Management of epilepsy in women of childbearing age; practical recommendations. CNS Drugs 20(5):373–387

Walsh M (ed) 2002 Watson's clinical nursing and related sciences, 6th edn. Bailliere Tindall, Edinburgh, p 739

Chapter 9

Diabetes mellitus

CHAPTER CONTENTS

INTRODUCTION

Diabetes mellitus is a chronic endocrine disorder of glucose metabolism. It results from defects in insulin production or action and is characterized by abnormal metabolism of carbohydrates, proteins and fats, which results in hyperglycaemia.

Diabetes mellitus is the most common of the endocrine disorders, and although the precise aetiology is still uncertain, environmental factors combine with a genetic susceptibility to determine which of those individuals actually develop the clinical syndrome and the timing of its onset.

There are three variations of diabetes relevant to pregnancy. Types 1 and 2 diabetes mellitus and gestational diabetes. The severity of these conditions varies and affects pregnancies to differing degrees. The midwife must have a good understanding of the pathophysiology of diabetes in order to recognize its presence and refer her client to the appropriate medical practitioner.

RELEVANT ANATOMY AND PHYSIOLOGY OF PANCREAS

The pancreas is an oblong gland, approximately 12.5 cm long and 2.5 cm thick. It is situated in the epigastric region posterior to the greater curvature of the stomach, and is connected by two ducts to the duodenum (Fig. 9.1). The head is the expanded portion situated near the 'C' shaped curve of the

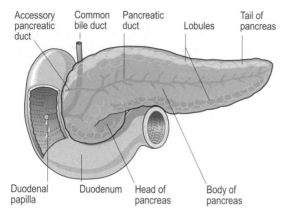

Figure 9.1   Gross anatomy of the pancreas.

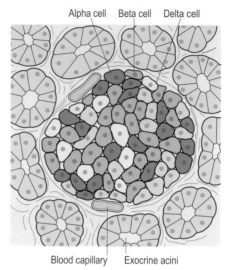

Figure 9.2   Islet of Langerhans.

duodenum, superior and to the left are the central body and tail.

The pancreas is both an endocrine and an exocrine gland. Endocrine glands secrete hormones into the blood, while exocrine glands secrete their products through ducts into body cavities or onto body surfaces. The largest portion of the pancreatic cell mass is composed of acini – clusters of cells which constitute the exocrine or digestive portion of the gland, secreting a mixture of digestive fluid and enzymes called pancreatic juice into the duct system. Pancreatic secretions pass from the secreting cells into ducts that ultimately convey the secretions into the small intestine.

Pancreatic juice is a clear, colourless fluid containing water, salts, sodium bicarbonate and enzymes which digest carbohydrate, fat and protein. The main enzymes involved in this process are amylase, lipase and trypsin. Normally, the amount secreted is approximately 1200–1500 mL/day in the adult.

Interspersed within the acini are small clusters of cells called the islets of Langerhans or pancreatic islets, which form the endocrine portion of the pancreas (Fig. 9.2). There are four types of cells within the islets, which secrete the following hormones:

- Alpha cells, which secrete glucagon
- Beta cells, which secrete insulin
- Delta cells, which secrete somatostatin
- 'F' cells, which secrete pancreatic polypeptide.

A brief synopsis of the endocrine function of the pancreas is provided to emphasize the importance of the pancreatic function in metabolic homeostasis.

Pancreatic polypeptide regulates the release of pancreatic digestive hormones. Somatostatin, or growth hormone inhibiting factor (GHIF), acts as a paracrine (a local hormone which acts on neighbouring cells), to inhibit the secretion of insulin and glucagon. Glucagon and insulin are the endocrine secretions of the pancreas and are concerned with the regulation of blood glucose.

If glucose is not required by the body immediately for energy, then it is converted to glycogen and stored in the liver and skeletal muscle. Glucagon acts mainly on the liver, and its principal activity is to increase the blood glucose level by accelerating the conversion of glycogen to glucose. This process is known as glycogenolysis. Glucagon also aids the conversion of other nutrients such as certain amino acids and lactic acid into glucose, known as gluconeogenesis. The liver then releases glucose into the bloodstream and the blood glucose level rises.

Secretion of glucagon is via a negative feedback system (Fig. 9.3); if the blood glucose level falls below normal, chemical sensors stimulate the alpha cells to secrete glucagon. When blood glucose level rises, the cells are no longer stimulated and production ceases. Exercise and protein-heavy meals also stimulate glucagon secretion. Somatostatin inhibits glucagon secretion.

Emotional stress commonly raises blood glucose levels. Cortisol is a corticosteroid hormone

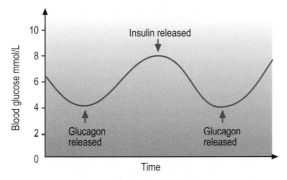

Figure 9.3   Control of blood glucose.

produced by the adrenal cortex and is involved in the response to stress. It increases blood pressure and blood glucose levels. Cortisol has widespread actions which help to restore homeostasis after stress. Cortisol acts as a physiological antagonist to insulin by promoting gluconeogenesis, the breakdown of fats and proteins and the mobilization of amino acids and ketone bodies. This leads to an increase in blood glucose levels and the storage of glycogen in the liver (Marieb & Hoehn 2007).

Insulin is produced by beta cells. Its physiological action is the reverse of glucagon. Insulin accelerates the transport of glucose from the blood into the cells, especially skeletal muscle cells, and thereby decreases the blood glucose level. Insulin also accelerates the conversion of glucose to glycogen. This is known as glycogenesis. It decreases glycogenolysis and gluconeogenesis and stimulates the conversion of glucose and other nutrients into fatty acids (lipogenesis). Insulin also stimulates protein synthesis.

Regulation of insulin is determined by the glucose level in the blood. Increased blood glucose levels stimulate insulin secretion, while decreased blood glucose levels inhibit it (Fig. 9.3). Increased levels of certain amino acids also stimulate insulin release. Human growth hormone (hGH) and adrenocorticotrophic hormone (ACTH) both raise blood glucose levels, and the rise in blood glucose level stimulates insulin secretion. Somatostatin inhibits the secretion of insulin.

Metabolism

The word 'metabolism' is translated from '*metabolismos*', the Greek word for 'change', or 'overthrow'.

Metabolism is the biochemical modification of chemical compounds in living organisms and cells. This includes the biosynthesis of complex organic molecules and their breakdown. Nutrients are digested and broken down into chemical compounds; some of these chemical compounds recombine to form other compounds or building blocks (anabolism) and some chemicals break down to provide energy (catabolism).

Metabolism usually consists of sequences of enzymatic steps, or metabolic pathways which are a series of chemical reactions occurring within a cell, catalyzed by enzymes. Many of these pathways are elaborate, and involve a step by step modification of the initial substance to shape it into the product with the exact chemical structure desired. Catabolic pathways break down complex molecules into simple compounds, while anabolic pathways create building blocks and compounds from simple precursors.

Carbohydrate metabolism

Carbohydrate metabolism is primarily concerned with glucose metabolism as glucose is the body's preferred source of energy.

When digesting foodstuffs, polysaccharides and disaccharides are hydrolyzed (broken down) to become monosaccharides; these are glucose, fructose and galactose.

To simplify, complex sugars are broken down to become simple sugars. These simple sugars are absorbed into the capillaries of the villae of the small intestine and transported to the liver via the portal vein where the majority of fructose and galactose is converted to glucose. If required, some glucose is oxidized by the cells to provide energy while the remaining glucose moves into cells by facilitated diffusion (a carrier protein makes the glucose soluble allowing it to pass through the selectively permeable cell membrane from a region of higher concentration to a region of lower concentration).The rate of glucose transport is greatly accelerated by insulin. Excess glucose can be stored by the liver and skeletal muscle as glycogen, or converted into fat and stored as adipose tissue. When required, glycogen can be converted back to glucose, which is then released into the bloodstream and transported to cells to be oxidized.

Fat metabolism

Lipids or fats are the body's second preferred source of energy, although more usually, fats are utilized as building blocks to form essential structures.

When lipids such as triglycerides are eaten, they are digested and hydrolyzed to become fatty acids and monoglycerides. Lipids are oxidized to produce energy, and produce more than twice the amount of energy than carbohydrates, but they are rather more difficult to catabolize than carbohydrates. If the body has no need for energy from lipid breakdown, then the fats can be stored as adipose tissue throughout the body, including the liver. Insulin stimulates fat synthesis and inhibits fat breakdown.

Protein metabolism

Proteins are broken down by the process of digestion into amino acids. They are absorbed by villi in the small intestine and transported in the bloodstream to the liver. Amino acids enter body cells by active transport (a process in which energy is used to move a chemical substance across a cellular membrane from a region of low concentration to a region of high concentration). Insulin stimulates the active transport of amino acids into cells, particularly muscle cells.

Summary   Nutrients may be oxidized for energy, converted into other molecules or they may be stored. Enzymes control the metabolic pathway of individual nutrients and hormones are the primary regulators of metabolism. Vitamins and minerals are necessary for effective hormonal control, and some of these are components of the enzymes, which serve as biological catalysts for specific molecules. Pancreatic juice and pancreatic hormones play a significant part in this process.

TYPES OF DIABETES MELLITUS

There are two main types of diabetes mellitus. Type 1, which was formerly known as insulin dependent diabetes mellitus (IDDM), occurs mainly in the young. Type 2, which was known as non-insulin dependent diabetes mellitus (NIDDM) was said to occur in the middle-aged, overweight adult. These are rather simplistic generalizations and not entirely accurate, as insulin may be required in individuals with type 2 diabetes mellitus and also type 2 diabetes is now occurring in younger age groups. Other forms of diabetes include impaired glucose regulation, which refers to a metabolic state between normal glucose homeostasis and diabetes. This condition may be a risk factor for the development of diabetes in the future. Maturity onset diabetes of the young (MODY) is a rare type of diabetes associated with genetic defects. For the midwife, this discussion will focus on the two main types of diabetes mellitus and the form of diabetes which occurs in pregnancy – gestational diabetes mellitus.

Type 1 diabetes mellitus

Aetiology

The aetiology of type 1 diabetes mellitus is thought to be multifactorial and far from being completely understood. It is considered to have an autoimmune basis and a number of risk factors have been identified, which may be divided into genetic and environmental. These risk factors include links to chromosomes and several chromosomal regions have been implicated. The most significant gene loci defining the risk of type 1 diabetes are to be found within leucocyte antigen (HLA) gene region (BMA 2004).

There has been a rapidly rising incidence in migrant populations suggesting environmental links, for example viral infections. It has been observed that IgM antibodies to Coxsackie B virus are found in 25–35% of newly diagnosed diabetics (Kanno et al 2006). An increased incidence of type 1 diabetes has been noted in individuals with congenital rubella, and cytomegalovirus DNA has also been found in 22% of newly diagnosed diabetics (Jaeckel et al 2002).

It has also been suggested that those with diabetes were breast-fed for a significantly shorter time than non-diabetic infants, and that the incidence of diabetes can be modified by the exclusion of cow's milk, suggesting that early exposure to cow's milk may be an important factor in the aetiology of type 1 diabetes (BMA 2004). The condition varies considerably in incidence between cultures with the 10 countries with the highest proportion of sufferers being India, China, USA, Indonesia, Japan, Pakistan, Russia, Brazil, Italy and Bangladesh (WHO 2006).

Incidence

The incidence of diabetes mellitus appears to be on the increase, and a likely factor related to this increase is obesity and lifestyle in western culture. The prevalence of diabetes for all age-groups worldwide was estimated to be 2.8% in 2000 and is estimated to rise to 4.4% by 2030 (Wild et al 2004). The total number of people with diabetes is projected to rise from 171 million in 2000 to 366 million in 2030.

The costs to people's quality of life, the economy, society and the NHS, are already evident. Diabetes can lead to serious complications, such as heart disease, blindness, kidney failure and stroke and nerve damage, leading to amputation (Diabetes UK 2006).

There are several reasons why the prevalence of diabetes is increasing: the greater life expectancy means that there is an increasingly ageing population. Also, the UK has a rapidly growing obesity problem, and the risk of developing type 2 diabetes increases by up to 10 times in people with a body mass index (BMI) >30. In people with an African-Caribbean or Asian background, the prevalence is approximately five times higher than that of the indigenous population (BMA 2004).

Signs and symptoms

Traditionally, type 1 diabetes is said to occur in the young with a rapid onset and severe clinical features including nausea, vomiting, malaise and fatigue.

Classically, the three 'polys' are described:

Polydipsia – excessive thirst
Polyuria   – excessive micturition
Polyphagia – voracious appetite.

Sudden weight loss, in spite of a good appetite may occur in severe forms. Glycosuria is characteristic and if combined with ketonuria in the absence of fasting, type 1 diabetes is suspected.

Pathophysiology

Type 1 diabetes mellitus occurs as the result of rapid and progressive loss of beta cells, resulting in an absolute deficiency of insulin, and is thought to be precipitated by a response to physical or psychological stress.

Lack of insulin has a domino effect, as cells cannot therefore obtain glucose for metabolism and this illustrates how the clinical features arise. Ingested glucose which is unable to enter cells accumulates in the blood leading to hyperglycaemia; this high blood glucose level circulates throughout the body including the renal system, which cannot cope with the increasing amounts of glucose. As a consequence, the renal threshold is exceeded, and glucose appears in the urine, resulting in glycosuria. Glucose is highly osmotic (it attracts and holds water to itself), therefore, as glucose is lost in the urine, large volumes of water are lost with it. This is known as polyuria. Furthermore, nocturia may occur resulting in disturbed sleep patterns. As fluid loss continues, symptoms of dehydration occur, resulting in copious drinking in response to severe thirst – polydipsia.

As the cell requirements for glucose are not being met, the response is for increased secretion of glucagon. Glycogen is converted back into glucose and released by the liver – glycogenolysis. However, glycogen storage is quickly depleted and in an attempt to supply the cells there is a breakdown of body fat and protein to produce glucose – gluconeogenesis.

Body cells are not being supplied with glucose, so may stimulate appetite – polyphagia, although this may be tempered somewhat because of nausea and/or vomiting. Weight loss occurs due to depletion of body fat and insulin stores, which together with cell deprivation of glucose, fluids and electrolyte imbalance results in muscle weakness and exhaustion. This exhaustion may be so overwhelming as to mask the presence of the other clinical features in the affected individual.

Because there is no insulin, fat metabolism results in ketone bodies being produced. These accumulate in the blood and urine, causing ketonaemia and ketonuria. Ketone bodies are weak acids, which release free hydrogen ions causing metabolic acidosis. Excess acidity in the blood causes hyperventilation – the body's response to removing excessive hydrogen ions.

Uncontrolled and untreated, these features will lead to a life-threatening condition known as diabetic ketoacidosis (McIntyre & Strachan 2000).

Diagnosis

Onset of type 1 diabetes mellitus is often sudden, but can vary in severity, with some patients acutely ill at the time of diagnosis. Sudden weight loss, thirst and passing frequent and large amounts of urine, particularly at night, with increasing tiredness is noted by the patient or their parents, causing them to visit their family doctor. The GP may perform urinalysis to test for glucose and ketones, although urinalysis is not an accurate or precise measure of high or low blood glucose levels. Blood glucose will also be measured, a normal blood glucose level is 4–7 mmol/L, and a result of 11.1 mmol/L or more in the symptomatic patient is indicative of diabetes mellitus.

Where symptoms are suggestive, but not conclusive of diabetes, a fasting blood glucose analysis will be carried out on 2 separate days, and a result of >8 mmol/L is indicative of diabetes mellitus.

Patients who are acutely ill at the time of diagnosis because of the rapid onset of the condition may be drowsy or semi-conscious due to diabetic ketoacidosis. These individuals will require urgent hospital admission to treat the acidosis and to stabilize their diabetes.

Hospital admission is not automatic. Currently, patients less acutely ill may be referred to diabetic day centres where full assessment may be carried out by a multidisciplinary diabetic team, including a diabetic consultant, specialist diabetic nurse practitioners, dieticians, ophthalmologist and podiatrists.

Management

The mainstay of care is dietary advice, insulin, blood glucose monitoring, education and psychological care. At the time of diagnosis, intensive educational and psychological support is provided and as the patient learns and becomes more familiar with the condition, she will be encouraged to manage her own condition. Newly diagnosed individuals may experience a wide range of emotions including shock, anger and fear. Because of this, education should be given in small bites and verbal information should be backed up with written reinforcement. Information on how to contact the diabetic liaison nurse by telephone or a local diabetic self-help group is also helpful.

Box 9.1 Administration of insulin

Insulin is available in different presentations depending on the device used. Insulin vials are used with insulin syringes. Insulin cartridges are used with reusable pens and disposable pre-filled pens are also available.

Insulin is administered by subcutaneous injection. There are three main areas for injection – abdomen, buttocks and thighs (Fig. 9.4). The upper arm is the least preferred site as it has little subcutaneous tissue. Overuse of one site can lead to fat hypertrophy and loss of sensitivity. If insulin is injected into fatty tissue, this will result in slower and more erratic absorption of insulin, resulting in variable and unstable blood glucose readings. It is advisable to use a different site each day and by rotating sites, this ensures the insulin will act quickly and effectively.

To reduce the discomfort of an injection, some newly diagnosed diabetics hold an ice cube against the skin for a few seconds, just prior to injection. This can help numb the area to any pain.

Giving insulin injections is usually a concern, and must be demonstrated and practised carefully by the individual until they feel confident. Alcohol swabbing is contraindicated, as it causes the skin to toughen, making injections more difficult. Needle length, angle of injection, as well as suitable sites for injection must also be addressed (Box 9.1, Fig. 9.4). Various devices are available to deliver insulin to the individual, including insulin pens, which are loaded with a single use cartridge containing the required dose.

On-going education is provided regarding the type of insulin used, how it works, and how to adjust the dose according to the patient's level of activity and blood glucose levels.

Capillary blood glucose monitoring is also demonstrated and practised until the individual feels proficient. Most newly diagnosed individuals choose to purchase a blood glucose meter (not available on prescription, although the test strips and lancets for use with the meter are available on prescription). Some diabetic nursing teams can supply glucose meters free of charge.

Glucose tests are usually carried out four times daily before meals and at bedtime and should aim to keep blood glucose levels between 4–7 mmol/L.

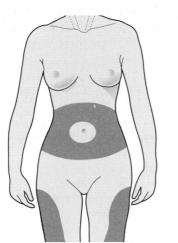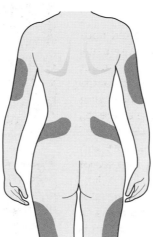

Figure 9.4   Sites of injection.

The advantage of daily blood glucose monitoring is that it provides day-to-day control and greater patient involvement in managing their diabetes.

Glycosylated haemoglobin (HbA$_{1c}$) is a valuable blood test which identifies the proportion of haemoglobin bound to glucose, and averages blood glucose levels over a 6–8 week period – the life span of a red blood cell – thereby providing an estimation of diabetic glycaemic control over this time. Ideally, the target of glycosylated haemoglobin is ≤7% for people with type 1 diabetes and between 6.5% and 7.5% for people with type 2 diabetes.

Urinalysis is not routinely carried out, as it is unhelpful for all those using insulin. It does not diagnose low blood glucose levels nor can it be used to identify a hypoglycaemic event. Furthermore, it is considered that urinalysis provides neither an accurate nor a precise measurement of high or low blood glucose levels (Diabetes UK 2006).

First aid dietary advice may be given by the nurse but mainly the dietician assesses the patient and provides individualized education. A healthy diet, which includes high levels of complex carbohydrate and fibre, moderate protein, and low fat, particularly saturated fats, is recommended. Regular meals, five portions of fruit and vegetables, plenty of water, avoiding sugary drinks and cakes and reducing salt intake will go far to ensure a healthy diet.

The most important issues are that the individual must be supported in this very difficult time and that she has access to specialist diabetic care resources and self-help groups. 'Buddy' support groups where an experienced diabetic teams up with a newly diagnosed individual are useful but must not replace professional support (Scottish Diabetes Framework 2006).

Insulin Insulin today is prepared from highly purified bovine (beef) or porcine (pig) insulin, which is more similar to human insulin; or biosynthetic human insulin, which has greatly reduced the adverse effects experienced by some patients on insulin therapy. There are various forms of insulin including soluble, isophane, insulin zinc suspension and biphasic insulins.

Short-acting insulins, e.g. soluble insulin, reach therapeutic levels 20–30 min after injection and peak 1.5–4 h post-injection. Analogue insulins enable immediate absorption following injection and may be administered immediately before eating or up to 15 min afterwards. Intermediate-acting insulins act about 1 h after injection and peak between 2 and 12 h depending on the specific insulin used. Duration of effect of these drugs is 18–24 h.

Long-acting insulins reach therapeutic levels 2–4 h after injection, peak between 4 and 24 h and last for up to 28 h.

Type 2 diabetes mellitus

The main factors associated with this type of diabetes are obesity, particularly central obesity, where the individual is described as 'apple-shaped', with a sedentary lifestyle, or if the individual is of South Asian or African-Caribbean origin or has a family history and is middle-aged (Diabetes UK 2006). There has however, been a significant increase in the number of younger people of child-bearing age who have developed type 2 diabetes, probably due to increasing obesity and lack of exercise (Scottish Diabetic Framework 2002).

Type 2 diabetes is significantly more prevalent in adults who had low birthweight for gestational age. Undernutrition in fetal life may result in per-manent physiological changes that would be ben-eficial if nutrition remained scarce after birth. But, if nutrition becomes plentiful, these changes pre-dispose to obesity and impaired glucose tolerance. This has been described as the thrifty phenotype hypothesis (BMA 2004).

In type 2 diabetes, the beta cells fail to produce adequate amounts of insulin in response to glucose from meals. Alternatively, tissue sensitivity to insu-lin may decline. This is known as insulin resistance and results in hyperglycaemia in spite of ade-quately circulating insulin. What must be stressed is that type 2 diabetes mellitus is not a milder or less important form of diabetes. Life-threatening complications can arise in this condition also. It is generally thought that a large percentage of people have sub-clinical diabetes and that there are nearly as many people with undiagnosed diabetes as there are diagnosed cases.

Clinical features

These are similar to type 1 diabetes but less marked due to a more gradual onset. Polyuria, thirst, and staphylococcal skin infection may present and cause the individual to seek medical help. Tiredness and exhaustion occurs insidiously, possibly due to an altered fluid and electro-lyte balance. Some individuals lose weight but many do not. Blurring of vision, due to the hyper-glycaemia, which causes opacity of the lens and dehydration of lens fluid may also occur. Because even a minute amount of insulin is still being pro-duced, ketogenesis is inhibited, and ketonuria does not occur.

Diagnosis is often made or suspected by the GP or practice nurse based on clinical features. Frequently, the condition is picked up by screening tests, such as those carried out at a well-woman clinic. However, if the presenting features are inconclusive, diagnosis may be made in the non-symptomatic individual, by a fasting blood glu-cose analysis carried out on 2 separate days, where results of >8 mmol/L are diagnostic.

Management

Management may be provided by the GP and prac-tice nurse or in some cases, the patient is referred to the diabetologist. Dietary advice and educa-tion are equally important in type 2 diabetes as in type 1. In March 2004, a structured group educa-tion programme was launched in order to integrate clinical care with education and self manage-ment. This programme aims to provide Diabetes Education and Self Management for Ongoing and Newly Diagnosed (DESMOND) people with type 2 diabetes; initially, this was piloted in England but is now spreading throughout the UK.

Management may be one of three combinations: diet alone, diet and oral hypoglycaemic agents, or diet and insulin. Initially, a 3-month period of diet and support by the practice nurse is provided. Oral hypoglycaemic drugs are required by up to 50% of individuals. There are several types that are used; some, but not all, are briefly described below.

- Sulphonylureas work by stimulating the pan-creas to produce insulin and are used in indi-viduals with some beta cell function. They reduce fasting blood glucose levels, but do not affect raised blood glucose following meals. These drugs may cause hyperinsulinaemia leading to weight gain. Examples include gliclazide and glibenclamide

- Biguanides decrease gluconeogenesis, which is the conversion of protein and fat to glucose. Additionally, they decrease the uptake of glu-cose by reducing the uptake of carbohydrate from the gut. These drugs are only used where there is some residual beta cell function and are not associated with weight gain. Metformin is the only biguanide available in the UK

- Alpha glucosidase inhibitors reduce blood glucose levels by delaying the digestion and absorption of glucose from the intestines.

There are other types of anti-diabetic drugs/oral hypoglycaemic agents available, but all women with type 2 diabetes will have to commence insulin therapy before or during pregnancy and when breast-feeding, as these drugs are contraindicated at these times.

Emergency complications of diabetes mellitus

Diabetic ketoacidosis   This is an acute complication of type 1 diabetes, and is the principal cause of diabetic related deaths in children and young adults. It may present at diagnosis, although, as early diagnosis becomes more common, this is less likely. Severe infection, acute illness or poorly managed diabetes with insufficient or missed insulin may also precipitate this complication.

Pathophysiology   Hyperglycaemia, gluconeogenesis and glycogenolysis lead to formation of excessive ketone bodies and this results in metabolic acidosis. Polyuria occurs as the kidneys attempt to reduce the blood glucose levels by excreting glucose in the urine, and despite drinking copious amounts of fluids, this leads to a worsening dehydration.

Nausea and vomiting may occur, possibly due to concurrent infection, and will exacerbate the dehydration causing electrolyte imbalance of sodium and potassium. In later stages, renal perfusion is reduced leading to decreased urinary output. Untreated, this results in decreased organ perfusion and function, and decreased oxygen delivery. These patients do not die of hyperglycaemia or lack of insulin – they die from hypoxia and hypovolaemia (Page and Hall 1999).

Clinical features   The patient may be unconscious, and a history may only be gleaned from relatives. On examination, there will be evidence of severe hyperglycaemia, polyuria and the individuals if conscious, will complain of extreme thirst. Clinically, there will be signs of dehydration, inelastic skin, dry mouth, sunken eyes, confusion and irritability. Tachycardia, due to the dehydration and hypovolaemia, and oliguria with ketonuria may also be present. Tachypnoea, deep, rapid, laboured respirations, will be observed and the breath will have a sweet fruity smell of acetone from the ketosis. Blurred vision caused by osmotic changes to the lens of the eye, may be present. Nausea and vomiting may occur and some individuals may complain of muscle cramps or abdominal pain, but it must be remembered that these may be features of underlying illness.

Management of diabetic ketoacidosis   The main aims of management directed by the diabetologist and diabetic team are to ensure an adequate airway and maintain breathing and circulation. The patient will be rehydrated via rapid i.v. infusion using isotonic fluids to restore intravascular volume and increase cardiac output. The electrolyte imbalance will be corrected in response to blood biochemistry, and hyperglycaemia reversed by administering rapid-acting insulin. Urine volumes will be monitored closely to identify renal damage (NICE 2004).

Although the ultimate responsibility is that of the diabetologist, the practitioner providing care must be meticulous in measuring and recording observations (Table 9.1).

Information and explanation must be given to both patient and relatives, and once initial emergency management has been provided, the patient's care will be transferred to the diabetic team for subsequent management to prevent recurrence.

Diabetic hyperglycaemic hyperosmolar coma or non-ketotic hyperglycaemic coma   This is a complication of type 2 diabetes that results in extremely severe hyperglycaemia without the presence of ketones. It mainly occurs in non-diagnosed type 2 diabetes and in an older age group (O'Hanlon-Nicholls 1996, cited in McIntyre and Strachan 2000).

Table 9.1   Observations in diabetic ketoacidosis

- Airway and breathing
- Level of consciousness
- Central venous pressure line as a guide to blood volume
- Monitor response to insulin therapy
- Assess capillary blood glucose hourly, venous blood glucose 2-hourly
- Blood pressure, temperature, pulse and respirations
- All fluid intake and output should be carefully and accurately recorded
- Exclude infection by blood cultures, urine specimen and throat swabs sent to laboratory, also sputum specimen when conscious

Serum osmolality is increased. In osmolar imbalances, there is a loss or gain of water affecting the concentration of the electrolytes, mainly sodium and potassium. In dehydration, there is water loss without a significant depletion of electrolytes, although there is an increase in the serum sodium level and osmolality. A hyperosmolar imbalance occurs when the blood is concentrated with sodium, glucose or other molecules which attract water into the bloodstream. Fluid therefore moves out of the cells into the circulation to maintain blood volume and consequently, the cells become dehydrated and have diminished function. The kidneys conserve body fluid by secreting less urine.

When body fluid is depleted, and osmolality increases, thirst occurs. If untreated, increasing dehydration occurs and concurrent diminished blood volume results in lowered blood pressure until the kidneys fail to excrete waste products and renal failure develops, which may result in death (Kitabchi et al 2001).

This is a serious metabolic complication, with significant hyperglycaemia, deficient insulin, severe dehydration and hypovolaemia. It may be precipitated by infection, undiagnosed or poorly managed diabetes, underlying kidney disease or by recent surgery. It may also occur in older people, particularly following myocardial infarction or cerebral vascular accident.

Immediate management directed by the diabetologist is similar to that of diabetic ketoacidosis (Table 9.2). Rehydration and intravenous insulin are tailored to the individual, and precipitating factors must be addressed. In addition, patients should receive DVT prophylaxis. Subsequent management should continue until all blood and biochemical levels are within normal limits.

Prior to discharge, patients should be reviewed by the diabetic team so that the cause of the coma can be established, education provided and review arranged.

Hypoglycaemia   This is an abnormally low blood glucose (<4 mmol/L) and can occur in both type 1 and type 2 diabetics. The individual will have taken her normal medication but some other factor such as missing out a meal or eating a meal with inadequate carbohydrate content, excess alcohol, or extreme exercise, may provoke a hypoglycaemic episode.

In addition, as hypoglycaemia is a common medical cause for accidents, the individual must be examined for other injuries (Bradley et al 2002).

Possible clinical features associated with blood glucose levels between 2.8–3.3 mmol/L include:

- Those due to adrenergic overactivity and include palpitations, pallor, sweating, nausea, tremor, anxiety and dilated pupils
- Those due to insufficient glucose to the CNS as the brain is dependent on a constant level of glucose for normal function. Any deprivation may seriously impair cerebral activity as indicated by hunger, disorientation and confusion, slurred speech, personality change, blurred or double vision, seizures and coma (Watkinson 2003).

Most individuals exhibit similar symptoms at each event of hypoglycaemia and thus will recognize the onset of the condition. Relatives and close friends should be familiar with these early signs and be instructed in the appropriate treatment.

Management   If the individual is conscious and cooperative, some form of rapidly acting source of sugar should be taken, for example, two teaspoonfuls of sugar, glass of milk, two digestive biscuits, Lucozade or Coca-Cola, followed by a long-acting carbohydrate such as a sandwich.

If the individual is unconscious, and providing venous access can be obtained, medical staff will usually prescribe 20–30 mL of 50% glucose i.v.,

Table 9.2   Midwifery observations in diabetic hyperglycaemic hyperosmolar coma

- Airway and breathing
- Level of consciousness
- Monitor ECG
- Oxygen saturation
- Intravenous access
- TPR
- Blood pressure
- Blood glucose, urea and electrolytes, serum bicarbonate and arterial blood gases

or alternatively, if venous access is not obtained 0.5 mg glucagon may be given i.m., and the patient monitored closely. Subsequent management will depend on the precipitating cause. A review of the individual's management of her diabetes may indicate some adjustment. The Diabetic Education Study Group produces leaflets for health professionals to use when educating patients on hypoglycaemia and other diabetic problems.

Prognosis The long-term complications of diabetes include atherosclerotic cardiovascular diseases, such as coronary artery disease, cerebrovascular accident (stroke) and peripheral vascular disease. Diabetes is one of the major aetiological factors in myocardial infarction, stroke and lower limb amputation. Cardiovascular disease accounts for 60% of all deaths from diabetes (BMA 2004). Diabetes is the fourth leading cause of death in the UK (Scottish Diabetes Framework 2002).

Additionally, diabetes damages small blood vessels resulting in changes to the microcirculation. These are reversible in the early stages but in the long term, in a poorly controlled diabetic, lead to considerable complications including diabetic retinopathy, nephropathy and neuropathy.

DIABETES IN PREGNANCY

Diabetes in pregnancy has long been recognized as a serious problem for both mother and fetus. Before the advent of insulin, women with diabetes rarely became pregnant; those who did, rarely carried the fetus to term. Although the outcome for pregnant women with diabetes has improved greatly over the last 50 years, Lindsay & Mackenzie (2006) concluded that stillbirth, perinatal mortality and congenital abnormalities remain between 2–5 times more frequent than in pregnancies not complicated by diabetes.

Even with good knowledge and management of diabetes nowadays, there remains an increased risk in both maternal and fetal morbidity and mortality. In the UK, diabetes complicates approximately 1% of all pregnancies in the Caucasian population and a higher percentage among other ethnic groups (Lloyd 2003).

Physiological changes in pregnancy

Pregnancy causes an increased insulin resistance, resulting in alterations in glucose metabolism and the stimulation of the beta cells of the pancreas to produce more insulin (Stables & Rankin 2005). Human placental lactogen (HPL), oestrogen and cortisol increase insulin resistance and alter carbohydrate tolerance; the net effect is to increase the availability of glucose and amino acid transfer to the fetus. In susceptible women, this may precipitate gestational diabetes. There has been some suggestion that a low glycaemic diet and exercise may help to minimize the increase in insulin resistance.

Effect of diabetes on pregnancy

Before insulin was available, maternal mortality was extremely variable and ranged from 6–50%. Currently, maternal mortality for women with diabetes is up to 43 times higher than for non-diabetic women (Hawthorne & Modder 2002).

Fertility is reduced in the woman with diabetes due to the progressive nature of the condition. However, many women with diabetes achieve normal pregnancies and births. There is, however, a higher incidence of complications, such as spontaneous abortion, stillbirth, and fetal abnormality (Lewis & Drife 2004, Lindsay & Mackenzie 2006). In addition, fetal macrosomia may lead to difficulties at the birth.

Pre-existing diabetes during pregnancy increases the risks both to the woman and the developing fetus. In addition to the physiological changes which normally occur in pregnancy, insulin requirements increase but vary with the individual (National Diabetic Support Team 2006). Poor diabetic control increases the severity of nausea and vomiting during the first trimester. Monilial and urinary tract infections are associated with hyperglycaemia.

The incidence of pre-existing diabetes, both type 1 and 2, has been estimated as 2–5% of the population of the UK (NICE 2004, Hawthorne & Modder 2002). Over half of the pregnancies complicated by diabetes involve gestational diabetes, although no exact figures are available.

All people with diabetes, whether type 1 or type 2 should be referred for preconception care

Box 9.2 Importance of preconception care in women with diabetes

Diabetes is the most common pre-existing medical disorder complicating pregnancy in the UK. Pregnancies complicated by diabetes mellitus, either pre-existing or appearing during pregnancy present an increased maternofetal risk. Good blood glucose control before and during pregnancy offers the best chance of reducing these risks. All healthcare professionals caring for diabetic women should advise them of the importance of preconception care. Preconception care should be provided by a multidisciplinary diabetic team. Women should be prescribed pre-pregnancy folic acid 5 mg daily and this should be continued up to 12 weeks' gestation.

(Box 9.2). Diabetic awareness sessions are a useful way of including people from ethnic minorities, as information can be delivered in different languages by interpreters in the wider local community. Advice provided should include planning a pregnancy and the use of effective contraception, particularly the use of barrier methods for 6 months prior to conception. A healthy diet and folic acid supplements should be recommended. A detailed review of their diabetes and lifestyle should be undertaken. Perhaps the most important part of preconception care is the communication by the health professional who provides it, for it is at this time that a relationship with the client is initiated and thus should lead to a professional partnership based on mutual trust and respect.

Optimization of glycaemic control before and during pregnancy reduces the incidence of congenital malformations, intrauterine death or stillbirth. The Confidential Enquiry into Maternal and Child Health (CEMACH 2005) recommends that blood glucose tests should be no higher than 5.5 mmol/L before meals and 7.7 mmol/L, 2 h after meals. Diabetic nurse specialists and midwives must provide explanations and information regarding the importance of accurate glucose monitoring, and should aim for targeting levels between 4–7 mmol/L.

Good glycaemic control can reduce the long-term progression of retinopathy and an eye examination should be carried out before conception by an ophthalmologist. This should be repeated during each trimester, as pregnancy can cause a rapid deterioration in diabetic retinopathy.

Pre-existing diabetic nephropathy must be closely monitored as proteinuria increases during pregnancy and this superimposed with pre-eclampsia is the most common cause of pre-term delivery. Hypertension is a condition commonly associated with diabetes, and substantially increases the risk of microvascular and macrovascular conditions, including stroke, cardiovascular disease and peripheral vascular disease, retinopathy and nephropathy. Hypertension must therefore be well controlled by the diabetologist. The antihypertensive agents suitable for use in pregnancy include methyldopa, labetalol or nifedipine. ACE inhibitors are contraindicated in pregnancy as they are hazardous to the fetus. Research has indicated that neural tube defects in high risk pregnancies are associated with lower levels of folate (SIGN 2001, Jincoe 2006). Folic acid 5 mg should therefore be commenced prior to conception and continued until at least 12 weeks' gestation.

During pregnancy, hypoglycaemia is common and diabetic ketoacidosis can develop more rapidly (SIGN 2001). Diabetic ketoacidosis is an obstetric emergency resulting in 50% fetal mortality and 5% maternal mortality. Untreated vomiting may lead to acidosis (Jordan 2002). Midwives must educate women and their families and friends on the prevention and management of both conditions. Verbal information should be reinforced with written leaflets. Emergency contact telephone numbers and arrangements must be explicit.

GESTATIONAL DIABETES

There is no consensus on the definition, management or treatment of gestational diabetes mellitus (GDM). GDM can be defined as carbohydrate intolerance of variable severity with onset or first recognition during pregnancy. This definition will include women with abnormal glucose tolerance that reverts to normal after delivery, and those with undiagnosed type 1 or type 2 diabetes.

Gestational diabetes is another name for carbohydrate intolerance of pregnancy. It occurs at around 20–24 weeks' gestation, when the placenta manufactures hormones (growth hormone and cortisol) that interfere with and block the body's ability to use insulin effectively, 'insulin resistance'. In an uncomplicated pregnancy, during the first trimester, blood glucose levels fall from 4 mmol/L to approximately 3.6 mmol/L and during the third trimester, fat stores laid down in the previous trimesters are utilized, with a resultant rise in free fatty acids and glycerol; the woman becomes ketotic more easily.

Resistance to insulin develops in all women during pregnancy, and in about 2–4% of women, this results in gestational diabetes. Insufficient insulin prevents glucose from entering body cells and effectively, these cells are starved of energy. The body then must convert protein and body fat into glucose for energy, resulting in the production of high levels of urea and ketones, which manifests as hyperglycaemia, ketonuria and proteinuria.

Certain women appear more likely to develop gestational diabetes, particularly if their history reveals one or more of the following:

- A family history of type 2 (adult-onset) diabetes
- Previous impaired glucose tolerance
- Hypertension
- Age <35 years
- Obesity
- Previous large baby
- Previous baby with an abnormality
- Previous intrauterine death late in pregnancy.

Diagnosis

Screening for GDM requires urine to be tested for glycosuria at every antenatal visit, and routinely at 28 weeks' gestation. As urinalysis is a routine part of normal midwifery care, this type of diabetes is often discovered at a routine antenatal visit where, if glycosuria is detected on two occasions, medical colleagues must be informed (NMC 2004). A random blood glucose specimen should be collected to determine the cause.

If the random blood glucose concentrations are not diagnostic but are >6.1 mmol/L in the fasting state or >2h after food, or >7.0 mmol/L within 2h of food, then an oral glucose tolerance test should be performed (Box 9.3). A diagnosis of gestational diabetes will be made if fasting blood

Box 9.3 Glucose tolerance test

Another method which may be employed to aid diagnosis is an oral glucose tolerance test (OGTT). The patient is fasted from midnight prior to the test. An initial blood glucose specimen is obtained before the patient is given 75g of glucose powder in 300 mL of water. A further blood glucose measurement is obtained after 2h. An elevated blood glucose level of 11.1 mmol/L or over, is diagnostic of diabetes mellitus (WHO 1999).

glucose is >7.0 mmol/L or >7.8 mmol/L 2h after a 75g glucose load.

Management of gestational diabetes

Women must be referred to diabetic and obstetric management, and care will be individualized and tailored to the individual woman, depending on her needs and diabetic control (SIGN 2001, CEMACH 2005). As well as the diabetologist and obstetrician, the multidisciplinary team will include the specialist diabetic nurse, dietician, podiatrist, physiotherapist and social services where necessary, as well as the midwife.

Dietary and lifestyle advice should be provided for all women. Small regular meals should be taken to ensure an adequate daily intake of low glycaemic index carbohydrates. Adequate calories and nutrients to meet the needs of pregnancy should be provided in the diet and should be consistent with the maternal blood glucose goals that have been established. For obese women, the dietician will devise with the woman, a calorie reduced diet with sufficient variety to reduce hyperglycaemia and plasma triglycerides without increasing ketonuria. The woman should also be encouraged to take appropriate exercise. Where fetal macrosomia is suspected, intensive dietary management and/or insulin therapy may be required.

Management of diabetes in pregnancy

Many of the initiatives started in preconception care are continued throughout pregnancy. Early contact by the midwife is desirable, as this will facilitate a professional partnership in care where the woman can receive appropriate education enabling her to make realistic informed choices. The midwife can also act as a liaison between other members of the team. As previously stated, diabetic pregnancies are high risk, and the clinical judgement of a diabetologist and obstetrician experienced in management of diabetic pregnancy is essential to reduce and manage complications (SIGN 2001). Antenatal assessment must be tailored to the individual; however, early referral as soon as pregnancy is confirmed is usual with 2-weekly visits until 28–30 weeks, and thereafter weekly until birth.

Regular ultrasound scanning will be offered to assess fetal size, gestational age and a detailed scan at 18–22 weeks to exclude fetal anomalies. Fetal monitoring may also involve regular cardiotocography and clinical assessment, particularly in the third trimester. Women should be alert for any perceived reduction in fetal movement and advised to contact the hospital when concerned.

CEMACH (2005) recommends that blood glucose levels should be maintained at no higher than 5.5 mmol/L before meals and 7.7 mmol/L, 2 h after meals. HbA$_{1c}$ should be less than 7%. Retinal assessment will be performed in early pregnancy to identify deterioration of function. Evaluation of renal function should also be undertaken. Constant review of medications will be required as pregnancy progresses and metabolic demands change.

The woman will be advised to give birth in an obstetric unit offering both high dependency facilities and a neonatal intensive care unit. If there are indications of pre-term labour, women should receive antenatal corticosteroid therapy according to local protocols. There is no clear evidence to inform the optimal timing of delivery, this must be determined on an individual basis, but the multidisciplinary team may advise induction between 37–39 weeks to prevent late intrauterine death. If fetal weight is estimated to be ⩾4.5 kg, an elective caesarean section may be considered.

Effect of pregnancy on diabetes

Nausea and vomiting in early pregnancy may upset diabetic control and lead to hypo/hyperglycaemia

(Taylor & Davison 2007). Tight glycaemic control is essential to prevent fetal morbidity. Initially, insulin requirements decrease, then increase between 18–28 weeks, gestation and dosage must be adjusted accordingly. Pregnancy may accelerate pre-existing retinopathy and/or nephropathy. There is an increased risk of severe hypoglycaemia.

Management of labour and birth

Normal diet and insulin are given prior to the onset of labour. Labour is likely to be induced with artificial rupture of membranes followed by oxytocin via infusion pump. During labour, intravenous dextrose 5%, 500 mL is infused 4-hourly, and insulin is given on a sliding scale to maintain blood glucose between 4–7 mmol/L. Capillary blood glucose levels are estimated hourly and insulin adjusted accordingly. Continuous fetal monitoring is undertaken because of the risk of fetal hypoxia, and a paediatrician will be present at delivery.

During the birthing process, the midwife should keep the woman and her family fully informed of the process and possible outcomes of the birth. As there is an increased risk of a large baby due to macrosomia (see below), the midwife should, wherever possible, allow the woman to adopt a birthing position other than the semi-recumbent position, to prevent compression of pelvic diameters. The multidisciplinary team will be alert for shoulder dystocia which occurs more frequently in the woman with diabetes and they will have well practised drills for dealing with such an event.

Puerperium

Postnatally, the mother's insulin requirements will fall rapidly, so close monitoring of blood glucose levels is mandatory; insulin dosage must be adjusted accordingly. In many units, the woman will remain on an i.v. infusion to allow venous access and prompt drug administration should it be necessary, until the woman's diabetic condition is stable and she is eating and drinking normally. Breast-feeding should be encouraged, but the woman must be supported in her choice of feeding method.

In breast-feeding mothers, insulin dose may be further reduced once lactation is established, but women with type 2 diabetes who are breast-feeding will usually need to continue with insulin (CEMACH 2005).

Education and support of women postnatally is vital and especially so in the early postnatal period where the woman may be in pain following operative delivery. Even after a spontaneous birth, she may feel very vulnerable due to the emotional strain of labour and birth. Continuity of care by the midwife is desirable for this woman, as a familiar midwife can be a source of comfort and understanding, particularly if emotional or social problems occur. With permission, the midwife will pass information to relevant team members. This facilitates supporting mechanisms to be put in place to sustain the woman and her baby in those first few weeks following birth. It is important to optimize communication and education through discussion and have it backed up by provision of written information; ideally telephone numbers should be provided to allow telephone consultations on days where home visits are not planned.

Postnatal follow-up should be seen as an opportunity to initiate pre-pregnancy care for a subsequent pregnancy. All women should be seen by the diabetes pregnancy care team 6 weeks after delivery. Women with gestational diabetes should be investigated postnatally to establish whether they had gestational diabetes or had in fact developed type 1 or type 2 diabetes. The opportunity should be taken to provide lifestyle advice, particularly on diet and exercise, in order to reduce the risk of subsequent type 2 diabetes.

Contraception should be discussed while the patient is still in hospital. All contraception carries some risk and each woman must be advised individually. Choice of contraceptive method will be discussed with the woman and her doctor who will advise her accordingly. The combined oral contraceptive pill with a low dose of oestrogen is safe for use in the majority of diabetic women. In some women however, a slight rise in blood pressure may be observed. The contraceptive pill may also raise cholesterol and triglycerides due to the effect of oestrogen contained in them. The progesterone-only contraceptive pill has the advantage of having a lesser effect on blood pressure or lipid metabolism. The failure rate of this pill is increased due to the need to take it at the same time every day to ensure contraceptive cover and this issue must be a consideration. Future pregnancies must be carefully planned to ensure optimal blood glucose levels at conception. Injectable and implantable progestogens are also suitable for some patients, particularly if compliance is an issue, although glycaemic control may deteriorate.

The main advantage of the intra-uterine contraceptive device is the lack of metabolic effects. Sterilization may be advised if further pregnancy represents a serious health risk.

Infants of mothers with diabetes

A paediatrician should be present at the birth of the infant of the diabetic mother due to the risks of fetal hypoxia and shoulder dystocia. However, most research suggests that it is unnecessary to routinely admit a baby to the neonatal unit (Bewley 2004). Whereas in the past these babies were often large and plethoric (Fig. 9.5), today with good glycaemic control, these infants are more likely to be appropriate for gestational age.

If the mother's diabetes is well controlled, and the baby is considered well and healthy

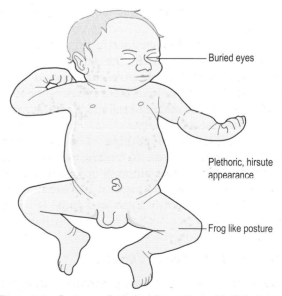

Figure 9.5   Features of a baby of a mother with diabetes.

Table 9.3   Risks to the baby of a mother with diabetes

Macrosomia	Excessive fetal growth – caused by uncontrolled maternal hyperglycaemia
Hypoglycaemia	Caused by hyperinsulinaemia due to hyperplasia of fetal beta cells because of maternal hyperglycaemia
Respiratory distress syndrome	Affects 10% of all premature infants. Caused by a lack of pulmonary surfactant, a complex material which reduces surface tension throughout the lung, thereby contributing to its general compliance
Polycythaemia	Caused by excessive erythropoiesis triggered by chronic fetal hypoxia
Hyperbilirubinaemia	Excessive red cell haemolysis commonly associated with polycythaemia leading to hyperviscosity
Hypocalcaemia	Due to failure to increase parathyroid hormone synthesis normally after birth
Congenital malformations	Due to increased perinatal survival and account for 30–50% of perinatal deaths. More common in poor glycaemic control
	Cardiac problems most common

following paediatric examination, then the infant should be admitted with the mother to the post-natal ward.

Poorly controlled diabetes often results in a macrosomic infant who may be physiologically immature. During pregnancy, increased maternal glucose levels affect fetal glucose homeostasis. As a result, beta-cell hyperplasia occurs in the fetal pancreas, stimulating an increase in release of insulin by the islets of Langerhans. Increased insulin levels stimulate fat and glycogen deposits and act as a growth factor resulting in fetal macrosomia. Following birth, the pancreas continues to produce excessive insulin but because the supply of glucose is no longer continuous after birth, the baby is at very real risk of developing hypoglycaemia.

Babies of mothers with diabetes must therefore be closely monitored. Early feeding will stimulate lactation and regular blood glucose estimation within 4h of birth, or sooner if the baby shows symptoms, will identify hypoglycaemia (Lewis & Drife 2004).

Neonatal hypoglycaemia is defined as a blood glucose <2.6mmol/L and is associated with adverse neurodevelopment. If borderline levels of blood glucose occur with ward testing they should be confirmed by laboratory testing, as research has questioned the accuracy of very low blood glucose levels with reagent sticks.

Other complications which may occur in the baby of the diabetic mother include respiratory distress syndrome (Table 9.3). Prior to birth, elevated insulin levels may inhibit the maturation of lung tissue by cortisol including the production of surfactant. This puts the fetus at risk for developing respiratory distress syndrome after birth. Jaundice caused by polycythaemia and weight loss may also occur and must be treated appropriately.

In conclusion, it can be seen that diabetes mellitus is a very complicated medical condition which can seriously affect pregnancy and childbirth. The woman must be the focus of care, which should be both sensitive and competent. Intra-professional cooperation, respect and liaison are of paramount importance, and a high standard of obstetric, medical and midwifery care is essential to ensure a successful outcome for the woman and her family.

REFERENCES

Bewley C 2004 Medical disorders of pregnancy. In: Henderson C, MacDonald S (eds) Mayes midwifery, 13th edn. Baillière Tindall, Edinburgh

Bradley K, Hammersley M, Levy J, Matthews D, Wallace T 2002 Guidelines for the management of hypoglycaemia. Oxford Centre for Diabetes, Endocrinology and Metabolism. Churchill Hospital, Oxford

British Medical Association (BMA) 2004 Diabetes mellitus – an update for healthcare professionals. Online. Available at: www.bma.org.uk/ap.nsf/Content/Diabetes (accessed February 2007)

Confidential Enquiry into Maternal and Child Health (CEMACH) 2005 Pregnancy in women with type 1 and type 2 diabetes in England, Wales and Northern Ireland. Executive Summary, London

Diabetes UK 2006 Online. Available at: www.diabetes.org.uk

Hawthorne G, Modder J 2002 Maternity services for women with diabetes in the UK. Diabetic Medicine 19(Suppl 1): 50–55

Jaeckel E, Manns M, von Herrath M 2002 Viruses and diabetes. Annals of the New York Academy of Science 958:7–25

Jincoe AB 2006 Diabetes: Monitoring maternal and fetal well-being. British Journal of Midwifery 14(2):91–94

Jordan S 2002 Pharmacology for midwives. Palgrave, Houndmills

Kanno T, Kim K, Kono K, Drescher K M, Chapman N M, Tracy S 2006 Group B coxsackie virus diabetogenic phenotype correlates with replication efficiency. Journal of Virology 80:5637–5643

Kitabchi A, Umpierrez G, Murphy M B et al 2001 Management of hyperglycaemic crises in patients with diabetes. (Technical review) Diabetes Care 24:131–135

Lindsay R S, Mackenzie F (2006) Diabetes and pregnancy. Journal of the Royal College of Physicians Edinburgh 36:312–314

Lewis G, Drife J (eds) 2004 Why Mothers Die 2000–2002: The sixth report of the Confidential Enquires into Maternal Deaths in the United Kingdom. RCOG, London

Lloyd C 2003 Common medical disorders associated with pregnancy. In: Fraser DM, Cooper MA (eds)

Myles textbook for midwives. Churchill Livingstone, Edinburgh, p 321–355

McIntyre R, Strachan 2000 Endocrine and metabolic disorders. In: Alexander M F, Fawcett J N, Runciman P J (eds) Nursing practice hospital and home: The adult. Churchill Livingstone, Edinburgh

Marieb E N, Hoehn K 2007 Human anatomy and physiology, 7th edn. Pearson Education, San Francisco

National Diabetes Support Team 2006 Fact sheet No. 21. Online. Available at: www.diabetes.nhs.uk

National Institute for Clinical Excellence (NICE) 2004 Type 1 diabetes: Diagnosis and management of type 1 diabetes in adults. Clinical Guidelines. NICE, London

Nursing and Midwifery Council 2004 Midwives rules and standards. NMC, London

Page S, Hall G 1999 Diabetes. Emergency and hospital management. BMJ Books, London

Scottish Diabetes Framework 2002 The Blueprint for Diabetes Care in Scotland in the 21st Century. Scottish Executive Health Department, Edinburgh

Scottish Diabetes Framework 2006 Action Plan: The Scottish Diabetic Buddy Service, Scottish Executive, Edinburgh

Stables D, Rankin J 2005 Physiology in childbearing, 2nd edn. Elsevier, Edinburgh

Taylor R, Davison J M 2007 Pregnancy plus. Type 1 diabetes and pregnancy. British Medical Journal 334:742–745

The Scottish Intercollegiate Guidelines Network (SIGN) 2001 Management of diabetes. SIGN Guideline 55. SIGN, Edinburgh

Wild S, Roglic G, Green A, Sicree R, King H 2004 Global prevalence of diabetes: Estimates for the year 2000 and projections for 2030. Diabetes Care 27(5):1047–1053

Watkinson M 2003 The practice of caring. In: Booker C, Nicol M (eds) Nursing adults. Elsevier, Edinburgh

WHO 1999 Definition, diagnosis and classification of diabetes mellitus and its complications: Report of a WHO Consultation, Part 1: Diagnosis and classification of diabetes mellitus. Department of Noncommunicable Disease Surveillance, World Health Organization, Geneva

WHO 2006 Fact Sheet No. 312. Diabetes. World Health Organization, Geneva

Chapter 10

Thyroid disorders

INTRODUCTION

Thyroid disease is one of the most common endocrine diseases likely to occur in women of childbearing age. Within the general population, thyroid disease is more likely to occur in the young adult woman, although both sexes may be affected. Thyroid disorders are among the most prevalent of medical conditions and increase with age. Overactivity, known as hyperthyroidism or thyrotoxicosis may be caused by a variety of disorders, for example, Graves' disease, thyroiditis, toxic multinodular goitre. Underactivity, known as hypothyroidism or myxoedema is considered to be an autoimmune disorder. Although normally already diagnosed and treated, the thyroid hormones may be affected by the process of childbirth and thus the midwife must have a clear knowledge of the implications for pregnancy, labour and the puerperium.

RELEVANT ANATOMY AND PHYSIOLOGY

The thyroid gland is an endocrine gland, responsible for producing, storing and secreting the thyroid hormones. The gland is located anteriorly to the trachea, just below the level of the thyroid cartilage, which forms the anterior surface of the larynx, and superior to the cricoid cartilage (Fig. 10.1).

The thyroid gland is shaped like a 'butterfly', having a right and left lobe joined by a narrow isthmus; normal weight in adults is 15–25 g.

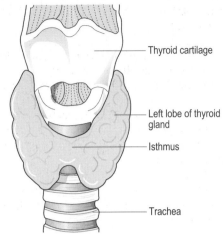

Figure 10.1   Anterior view of the thyroid gland.

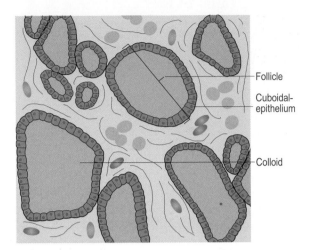

Figure 10.3   Microstructure of thyroid tissue.

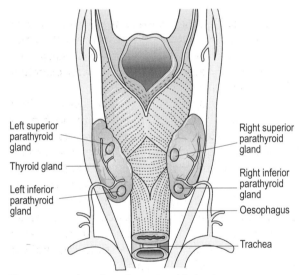

Figure 10.2   Location of parathyroid glands.

The thyroid gland has an extensive blood supply from the superior and inferior thyroid arteries, which are branches of the subclavian and external carotid arteries. Venous blood drains into three veins – superior and middle thyroid veins drain into the internal jugular vein. The inferior thyroid veins anastomose with each other and drain into the left brachiocephalic vein in the thorax. Four parathyroid glands are located behind the thyroid gland on its posterior aspect (Fig. 10.2)

Each lobe of the gland is divided into follicles, and each follicle is lined with a single spherical layer of cuboidal epithelium, surrounding a noncellular centre. The central follicular cavity contains a viscous gelatinous protein type material in suspension, referred to as a colloid (Fig. 10.3).

The glycoprotein that is secreted by the follicular cells is known as thyroglobulin. Iodine circulating in the bloodstream is removed and follicular cells trap and oxidize the element. At the apical surface of each follicular cell iodide ions are converted to an activated form of iodide (I^+) by the enzyme thyroid peroxidase.

Simultaneously, one or two iodide ions are attached to tyrosine molecules in thyroglobulin. Tyrosine–iodide ion molecules are paired forming molecules of thyroid hormones, resulting in the formation of the hormone thyroxine, T_4 containing 4 iodide ions, and the hormone tri-iodothyronine, or T_3 containing 3 ions (Martini 2005).

Thyroid hormones are released in response to hormonal signals from the hypothalamus and pituitary gland. Thyrotrophin releasing hormone (TRH) is secreted into the blood in response to low circulating concentrations of thyroid hormones. This in turn acts on the anterior pituitary which stimulates the secretion of thyroid stimulating hormone (TSH) and as the concentration of thyroid hormones rise, the production rates of TRH and TSH decrease. Therefore, the release of thyroid hormones is controlled by the level of thyroid stimulating hormone in the blood, and control is by a negative feedback system (Box 10.1).

The levels of T_4 (thyroxine) and T_3 (tri-iodothyronine) circulating in the blood are quite different. The thyroid gland makes more T_4 than T_3, and T_4

Box 10.1 Negative feedback systems

Feedback systems are essential within the body to ensure a constant supply of components vital to physiology such as hormones, blood sugar levels, etc. A feedback system is any circular situation in which information regarding the status of something is fed back to a central point. In the human body, the central point is commonly the central nervous system.

The most common feedback system in the body is a negative feedback system. A substance is released from a gland in response to a stimulus from the brain. Once this substance reaches a certain level, this information is fed back to the brain which then turns off the original stimulus. In the case of the thyroid gland low levels of thyroid hormones are detected by the hypothalamus which stimulates the pituitary gland via thyroid releasing hormone (TRH) to release thyroid stimulating hormone. Thyroid hormone levels rise and as they reach normal levels, TRH is inhibited.

One of the few positive feedback systems is seen in childbirth. Oxytocin is released from the hypothalamus via the pituitary gland and stimulates uterine contractions. As the cervix becomes dilated, this information is fed back to the hypothalamus, which releases increasing levels of oxytocin. This cycle is only interrupted by birth.

Table 10.1   Effects of thyroid hormones on body organs and tissues

- Increases the heart rate and force of the contraction, promoting normal function of the heart
- Promotes normal adult nervous system function; enhances the effects of the sympathetic nervous system
- Maintains normal sensitivity of respiratory centres to changes in oxygen and carbon dioxide concentrations
- Stimulates the formation of red blood cells and thereby enhances oxygen delivery
- Stimulates the activity of other endocrine tissues
- Accelerates the utilization of minerals in bones
- Regulates metabolic rate and heat production through glucose oxidization

Marieb & Hoehn 2007, Martini 2005, Jordan 2002.

has a longer half-life, but significantly, T_4 is less active and is used more as a storage form. In the peripheral circulation and at cell level T_4 can be converted to T_3 (de Swiet et al 2002).

Most of the thyroid hormones entering the bloodstream become attached to thyroid binding globulins, and only very small amounts remain unbound and are free to diffuse into peripheral tissues. Thyroid hormones readily cross cell membranes and they activate receptors involved with energy transformation and utilization; in other words, they regulate the metabolism of nearly all body cells. The critical effects from a midwifery perspective are that the thyroid hormones regulate carbohydrate, lipid and protein metabolism and the normal development of the nervous system in fetus and infant. They also promote normal growth and the hydration and secretory activity of the skin (Table 10.1). Female reproduction and lactation are also influenced (Marieb & Hoehn 2007).

Other larger endocrine cells are also found within the thyroid gland interspersed between the follicle cells. These are known as para-follicular or clear cells and produce the hormone calcitonin, which combined with parathyroid hormones coordinates the storage, absorption and excretion of calcium ions and phosphorus.

Calcitonin acts primarily on bone. Bone is in a constant state of remodelling, whereby old bone is removed by osteoclasts, and new bone is laid down by osteoblasts. Calcitonin inhibits bone removal by osteoclasts, and promotes bone formation by osteoblasts. In the kidney, calcium and phosphorus are conserved by reabsorption in the kidney tubules. Calcitonin inhibits tubular reabsorption of these two ions, leading to increased rates of their loss in urine. Thus, calcium ion balance is also maintained by a negative feedback system.

THYROID DISORDERS

Incidence

Thyroid disease is common in the general population and prevalence increases with age. Hypothyroidism is by far the most common disorder and is more common in older women. It is frequently the result of autoimmune disease, or may arise following radioactive iodine therapy or thyroid surgery for hyperthyroidism. Hyperthyroidism is much less common, with a female to male ratio of 9:1. Graves' disease is the most common cause and mainly affects young adults. Toxic multinodular goitres tend to affect older age groups.

Aetiology of thyroid disease

Hyperthyroidism

Graves' disease   This is the most common cause of hyperthyroidism. It is thought to be an autoimmune disease triggered by an infection or other stressor which leads to destruction of thyroid cells in susceptible individuals. It predominately affects females between 20–50 years, but can affect both sexes at any age. It is characterized by an enlargement of the gland (goitre) and ophthalmic features, e.g. lid-lag, lid-retraction with limited upward gaze (staring), exophthalmia, and retro-orbital inflammation leading to periorbital oedema.

Thyroiditis   This is rare condition, often referred to as subacute thyroiditis as frequently it occurs as a result of an upper respiratory tract infection. It is thought to be the major cause of pain in the thyroid gland. It can also present in patients taking the drugs interferon and amiodarone, a drug used in the treatment of some cardiac arrhythmias. Thyroiditis causes either a slow and chronic cell destruction, causing hypothyroidism, or conversely rapid cell destruction. If rapid cell destruction occurs, it produces symptoms of hyperthyroidism.

Toxic multinodular goitre   This type of goitre is characterized by an enlarged gland with distinct nodules. It tends to occur in an older age group outwith childbearing age.

Toxic adenoma (single nodule)   Toxic adenoma of the thyroid is an autonomously functioning thyroid nodule that produces excessive amounts of thyroid hormone leading to increased serum levels of T_3 and/or T_4 and suppression of serum TSH. The normal thyroid tissue that surrounds the nodule is often suppressed.

Pathophysiology

Excessive thyroid hormones produce signs and symptoms caused by an increase in the metabolic rate resulting in a variety of symptoms (Table 10.2).

Diagnosis

Clinical examination is confirmed by laboratory measurements of thyroid hormones. Both T_4 (thyroxine) and T_3 (tri-iodothyronine) levels are elevated but TSH (thyroid stimulating hormone) is almost undetectable. Ultrasound scanning is also used in the diagnosis of this condition.

Management

There are three approaches to treatment of this condition.

Antithyroid drug therapy   These drugs are prescribed to inhibit the synthesis of thyroid hormones. Carbimazole is the most commonly used drug, in dosages of 30–40 mg/day. If patients are sensitive to carbimazole, another drug which may be prescribed is propylthiouracil, 300–600 mg daily. The patient continues this therapy until a euthyroid state is achieved, then a maintenance dose is prescribed for approximately 1 year. Monitoring of the patient by her GP continues as required.

Rare but major possible side-effects of carbimazole are agranulocytosis (a partial or complete absence of neutrophils), or pancytopenia (deficiency in all blood cells) due to suppression of bone marrow function; and patients must be advised that if they develop a sore throat or unexplained fever, they must immediately seek medical advice.

Surgery   Partial thyroidectomy is only performed after the patient has achieved a euthyroid state and is useful if there is a large or unsightly goitre. Oral potassium iodide may occasionally be prescribed 1–2 weeks prior to surgery to reduce thyroid size and vascularity and inhibit thyroid hormone release, thereby reducing the risk of postoperative haemorrhage (Watkinson 2003).

Table 10.2   Symptoms of hyperthyroidism

- Heat intolerance, excessive sweating
- Irritability and restlessness
- Weight loss, despite increased appetite
- Diarrhoea
- Tachycardia, palpitations
- Atrial fibrillation, angina
- Dyspnoea
- Fatigue but difficulty in sleeping
- Weak muscles, difficulty in getting up from a squatting position
- Fine tremor of hands
- Amenorrhoea and infertility

Radioactive iodine therapy Radioactive iodine, iodine 131, may be used to treat hyperthyroidism. It is given orally in a single dose at an outpatient clinic. It acts by destroying follicular cells or inhibiting the cells' ability to replicate. Patients are advised that eating should be avoided for at least 4 h after administration of the isotope. This is to allow the drug to be absorbed adequately. Following this, the patient should drink at least 2 L of fluid over 24 h in order to excrete the free radioactive iodine as quickly as possible. This treatment is not usually offered to women of childbearing age (Dibbs 2001).

Whichever treatment is prescribed for the treatment of hyperthyroidism the patient will be anxious, due not only to her condition, but also due to the risks of each treatment. Careful explanation of the method of administration of drugs, and their risks must be given.

If operative treatment is prescribed, the patient is usually admitted prior to surgery for demonstration of postoperative physiotherapy. Information regarding the procedure should be provided to ensure they have understood medical explanations.

Thyroid cancer

Cancer of the thyroid gland is rare. Most nodules in the thyroid turn out to be benign. However, it tends to occur in a much younger age group than other malignancies. Surgery may be performed if necessary during pregnancy. With modern treatments now available, the outlook for people with cancer of the thyroid is very good and many people are completely cured.

Hypothyroidism

Underactivity of the thyroid gland may be primary, due to thyroid disease, or secondary due to pituitary failure. When there are insufficient circulating thyroid hormones hypothyroidism or myxoedema occurs. It is almost six times more common in women than men (Dibbs 2001, Perry 2003).

Primary hypothyroidism Primary hypothyroidism accounts for almost 95% of all cases of disease and is autoimmune in nature (Heuston 2001). It is often termed Hashimoto's disease or Hashimoto's thyroiditis and may be associated with other

autoimmune diseases, e.g. pernicious anaemia. In addition, there may be a family history of the condition. The development of microsomal autoantibodies leads to eventual atrophy and fibrosis of the gland (Kumar & Clark 2002).

Previous thyroid surgery or treatment by radioactive iodine for thyrotoxicosis can also lead to hypothyroidism, resulting in the need for lifelong thyroxine replacement therapy (Perry 2003).

Iodine deficiency is also another cause of hypothyroidism, due to insufficient dietary intake of iodine, leading to reduced thyroid hormone production.

Secondary hypothyroidism Secondary hypothyroidism occurs as a result of damage to the pituitary or hypothalamus, due to tumours, surgery or trauma, causing the synthesis of TSH to be impaired (Watkinson 2003).

Box 10.2 describes Derbyshire neck, a condition resulting from lack of iodine in the diet.

Box 10.2 Derbyshire neck

Endemic goitre was prevalent in the population of Derbyshire in the UK for many centuries until it declined from the 1930s. People thought that this was because Derbyshire was a long way from the sea where iodine was abundant in seafood. Recent research suggests the chemistry of the limestone environment seems to indirectly prevent iodine from entering the food chain (Fordyce 2002).

Goitre may occur if the thyroid gland is overactive, as in Graves' disease, or if underactive where dietary iodine is severely reduced, and the pituitary gland will sense the imbalance and produce more TSH. The thyroid gland will enlarge enough to make sufficient thyroxine. Goitre may occur without disease particularly in young women or during pregnancy. All goitres should be investigated because of the risk of malignancy (Marshall 1999).

According to the World Health Organization, iodine deficiency is the major cause of preventable mental retardation in the world today, with 1.6 billion people at risk, 50 million children affected and 100 000 sufferers born every year. Iodine deficiency disorders (IDD) have been halved and progress has been dramatic since the primary intervention strategy for IDD control – universal salt iodization – was adopted in 1993.

Table 10.3   Symptoms of hypothyroidism

- Periorbital puffiness
- Dull facial expressions and a low-pitched and hoarse voice
- Hair may be scanty, coarse and brittle
- Eyebrows are greatly thinned or even partly missing.
- Skin is often dry and scaly, cold, thickened and coarse
- Slowed in body and mind
- Depressed
- Decreased sweating
- Lethargic and easily fatigued
- Sensitive to cold
- Muscle pain (myalgia), slow reflexes paraesthesia
- Constipation
- Weight gain
- Menorrhagia or oligomenorrhoea

Clinical features The clinical features can be mainly attributed to a slowing down of body functions (Table 10.3). The onset is slow and the patient may be present with any of the clinical features listed, or if they have Hashimoto's disease, with a goitre.

Diagnosis Diagnosis will be confirmed by a raised thyroid stimulating hormone (TSH) and low or normal free thyroxine (T_4).

Treatment Hypothyroidism is treated with levothyroxine (thyroxine), usually commencing at a dose of 50–100 µg daily. The dose is gradually increased, and to ensure the patient is euthyroid both TSH and free T_4 levels are monitored. The aim is to provide sufficient levothyroxine to reduce the TSH to the lower level of normal and to raise the level of free T_4 to the upper half of the normal range (Perry 2003).

PHYSIOLOGICAL CHANGES IN PREGNANCY

During early pregnancy, TSH is slightly reduced, and then recovers as pregnancy continues. Thyroid hormones are normally unaltered, but from 12–14 weeks, there is an increase in the concentration of the plasma protein, thyroid-binding globulin (TBG) probably influenced by reduced hepatic clearance and oestrogen stimulation. Increased levels of TBG lead to lowered free thyroxine (T_4) concentrations, which results in elevated TSH secretion by the pituitary and, consequently, enhanced production and secretion of thyroid hormones. A balance is thought to be achieved by alteration in the metabolism of iodine. Renal iodide clearance doubles, plasma inorganic iodide falls and thyroid clearance of iodide trebles (Kettyle & Arky 1998).

Basal metabolic rate is thought to increase by approximately one-quarter from 4 months (Stables & Rankin 2005). Pregnancy therefore, results in an increased demand on the thyroid gland, which is easily met in the normal population, but in women with sub-clinical hypothyroidism pregnancy may precipitate clinical disease.

Toft (2004) suggests that chorionic gonadotrophin has a weak thyroid stimulating effect, therefore serum free thyroxine concentrations may increase and TSH concentrations may fall, resulting in a gestational thyrotoxicosis in a small number of women. This stance is also held by Kettyle and Arky (1998) stating that thyroid function remains normal during pregnancy although some women exhibit the signs associated with an overactive thyroid gland including thyroid hyperplasia or goitre.

Thyroid function tests in pregnancy

These blood tests are only undertaken when clinical examination suggests an abnormality, or if there is a family history of thyroid disease. Within the UK, it is not considered feasible to screen all pregnant women due to the effect of chorionic gonadotrophin which may make interpretation of TSH inaccurate (Pop et al 1999).

There are two forms of thyroid hormones, those that are bound to plasma proteins and act as a storage reservoir and those that are free. It is only the free hormones which are biologically active. In pregnancy, goitres may be physiological, and normal levels of thyroid hormones are altered. When obtaining blood specimens for thyroid function tests (Table 10.4):

- It should be stated clearly on laboratory forms that the woman is pregnant
- Record all medications prescribed; some may interfere with blood test

Table 10.4   Diagnostic thyroid function tests. Normal values

Test	Non-pregnant	Pregnant
Free serum thyroxine (T$_4$)	10–27 pmol/L	3rd trimester, 7–15 pmol/L
Total serum thyroxine (T$_4$)	64–142 nmol/L	64–256 nmol/L
Thyroid stimulating hormone	0.15–3.15 mU/L	1st & 2nd trimester 0.15–1.8 mU/L 3rd trimester 0.7–7.3 mU/L
Free serum tri-iodothyronine (T$_3$)	4–9 pmol/l	3rd trimester, 3–5 pmol/L
Total serum tri-iodothyronine (T$_3$)	1.0–2.6 pmol/L	1.0–2.6 pmol/L
Thyroid antibody test	Presence suggests	Hashimoto's thyroiditis

Jordan 2002.

- Thyroid medications; dose and time must be noted
- Free hormone concentrations must be requested.

Hyperthyroidism in pregnancy

Overactivity of the thyroid gland results in thyrotoxicosis and occurs in 0.2% of pregnancies (Schroeder 2002, Lazarus & Premawardhana 2005). Graves' disease is by far the most common cause of hyperthyroidism. This is an autoimmune disease characterized by antibodies in the circulation stimulating the production of thyroid hormones. Other causes of thyrotoxicosis include toxic multinodular goitre, toxic adenoma and subacute thyroiditis (Marshall 1999). Amiodarone, a drug used in treatment of cardiac arrhythmias can lead to the development of an overactive or underactive thyroid glad (Tan & Hurel 2001).

Signs and symptoms

Clinical features include a diffuse enlargement or goitre of the thyroid gland, raised BMR, with resultant diarrhoea and rapid weight loss in spite of a good appetite. Tachycardia and palpitations are common. The woman will complain of feeling excessively hot and will perspire copiously. Exophthalmos (protruding eyes), eyelid lag, pretibial myxoedema (skin thickening of the shins) and acropachy (swelling of the fingertips) may be evident. It is a relatively common disorder, which can occur at any age. Severe hyperthyroidism is associated with infertility but if the condition is mild pregnancy may be successful due to the increase of thyroid-binding globulin.

Diagnosis

Hyperthyroidism is difficult to diagnose in pregnancy because of normal pregnancy changes in thyroid function, but clinical examination and blood analysis will show evidence of raised T$_3$ and T$_4$ and decreased TSH and these will aid the physician in diagnosis. The thyroid gland may enlarge slightly in pregnancy, but even a moderately enlarged gland deserves investigation. This condition develops insidiously, and most patients have had symptoms for at least 3–6 months before presentation.

Management

Combined care by an endocrinologist and obstetrician is required, as this is a high risk pregnancy. Propylthiouracil or carbimazole are the most commonly used drugs and the levels and effects must be monitored closely. Full thyroid function tests must be reviewed frequently. The dietician will advise on nutrition to ensure a balanced diet with sufficient fluid and calorie intake to combat the increased metabolism and perhaps diarrhoea.

Hyperthyroidism must be adequately managed to reduce the risk for women of spontaneous abortion, pre-eclampsia, pre-term birth, or heart failure (Lazarus 2004). The goal is to control the hyperthyroidism and then use the lowest medication dose possible to maintain the serum thyroid hormone levels within the normal range.

In this way, smaller doses of medications are used, reducing the risk to the fetus.

If optimum control is difficult or if a women has a large goitre, then a sub-total thyroidectomy may be considered. This is usually performed in the mid-trimester (Becks & Burrow 2000).

Midwifery care should be of the normal high standard and must be woman centred. Women should be advised to have adequate rest, which they may find difficult to do, because of their condition. Careful questioning to ensure the woman is having sufficient sleep is also advisable. In an effort to minimize the incidence of infection during pregnancy, the woman should also be advised to avoid crowds. Labour and delivery are usually unaffected but, very occasionally, may be complicated with a thyroid storm.

Thyroid storm

This condition, also referred to as thyrotoxic crisis, is an acute, life-threatening, hypermetabolic state induced by excessive release of thyroid hormones in individuals with thyrotoxicosis. It is characterized by hyperpyrexia, severe vomiting, diarrhoea and extreme tachycardia.

Management of this serious condition should be in an ICU setting, with close monitoring of vital signs to enable access for invasive monitoring, with oxygen, ventilatory support and intravenous fluids to effect initial stabilization and management. There is a high rate of maternal morbidity and mortality with this condition.

Postnatal management of hyperthyroidism

During the third trimester of pregnancy, drug dosages can often be reduced, but thyroid levels must continue to be closely monitored. Soon after birth, thyroid levels will again rise and drug therapy will need increasing once again.

Effect of hyperthyroidism on the fetus

The human fetus starts to synthesize thyroid hormones at 10–12 weeks' gestation and thyroid hormones are necessary for fetal brain development. Perinatal mortality is high in untreated thyrotoxicosis, but can be reduced with adequate management. Treatment of Graves' disease by an antithyroid drug such as propylthiouracil blocks the production of thyroid hormones and thus may result in fetal or neonatal thyrotoxicosis.

Antithyroid drugs cross the placenta and fetal hypothyroidism is a definite risk with all antithyroid treatment, therefore the lowest possible maternal dose is given, sometimes leaving the woman in a slightly hyperthyroid state (Becks & Burrow 2000).

Fetal and neonatal hyperthyroidism may also occur. This is due to transplacental passage of maternal IgG thyroid stimulating immunoglobulins. Fetal hyperthyroidism is considered probable if there is fetal tachycardia (>160 beats/min) after 22 weeks' gestation. Untreated, the condition is associated with intrauterine growth restriction, craniosynostosis (a condition in which the sutures close too early, causing problems with normal brain and skull growth), or even fetal death. Dosage of maternal antithyroid drugs is altered to ensure the fetal heart rate is maintained at about 140 beats/min.

In neonates, vomiting, poor weight gain and hyperactivity occur and fetal condition may be complicated by cardiac failure or arrhythmias, or jaundice with enlarged spleen and liver. Neonatal management includes administration of iodine, dexamethasone, and sedation. Short-term management with antithyroid drugs may be life saving. The condition is often self-limiting, since the maternal immunoglobulins have a half-life of about 3 weeks in the infant.

Breast-feeding

There is some controversy regarding breast-feeding and hyperthyroidism, however, research indicates that propylthiouracil is the preferred drug when breast-feeding, as it is excreted to a lesser extent in breast milk than carbimazole (Marshall 1999). The infant's development and thyroid function should be supervised and monitored by a paediatrician (BNF 2005).

Hypothyroidism in pregnancy

In the UK, hypothyroidism is a fairly common condition occurring mainly in women and increasingly with age. Primary hypothyroidism accounts for the majority of all cases (Heuston 2001). It is an autoimmune condition where the development of antibodies leads to atrophy and fibrosis of the thyroid gland.

Another autoimmune manifestation is Hashimoto's thyroiditis, which also atrophies but the gland tries to regenerate the damaged tissue leading to goitre formation (Perry 2003). Other autoimmune diseases may also be present, such as diabetes mellitus or pernicious anaemia.

The treatment of an overactive thyroid gland by surgery or by radioactive iodine can also lead to hypothyroid disease, resulting in the need for life-long thyroxine replacement therapy. Rare causes of hypothyroidism include development of the condition secondary to hypothalamic or pituitary disorders, possibly following intracranial irradiation or surgical removal of a pituitary adenoma.

Signs and symptoms of hypothyroidism in pregnancy

In the UK, even very poor diets contain sufficient iodine for metabolic need, but in some other countries there is the risk of iodine deficiency. In many instances, individuals may attribute symptoms of hypothyroidism to life stresses and the diagnosis is made by the clinician. The individual may present with a vague feeling of being below par, feeling tired, lacking concentration. She may also be tearful or depressed, feeling very cold and there may be signs of a slowed metabolism, such as constipation or often, weight gain.

Diagnosis

The provisional diagnosis is usually made from clinical examination by the medical practitioner or practice nurse and is confirmed by blood analysis. The serum TSH is elevated and free thyroxine (FT_4) and free tri-iodothyronine (FT_3) may be below normal. A lipid profile may indicate hyperlipidaemia, which may resolve when the thyroid gland has returned to normal function, i.e. becomes biochemically euthyroid.

Management of hypothyroidism

Levothyroxine (thyroxine) is the drug used to treat hypothyroidism in pregnancy. It is commenced at a low dose of 50–100 µg daily and dosage is adjusted gradually in response to blood levels. The serum TSH level is a reliable indicator of need for dosage adjustment, and free thyroxine (FT_4) will confirm concordance. It would be prudent for the woman to attend for preconception care to ensure that her thyroid function is within normal range prior to pregnancy. All women with hypothyroidism should be advised to book early for antenatal care.

Women with hypothyroidism in pregnancy should be cared for by an endocrinologist and an obstetrician. Those who are well controlled may require fewer visits than those whose condition is less stable. Visits will therefore be tailored to the individual woman. Midwifery care should be directed towards forming a professional relationship where education and information giving is facilitated. Liaison with other members of the multidisciplinary team is essential to avoid duplication of visits.

Inadequate management of hypothyroidism in pregnancy is associated with an increased rate of spontaneous abortion, fetal death, congenital anomalies and pre-term delivery. Wolfberg et al (2005) found that women with hypothyroidism, which was adequately treated did not have an increased rate of fetal anomalies or preterm birth, although they did find a slightly higher rate of pre-eclampsia and small for gestational age infants born to these women, but noted that their finding were considerably less than previous reports. They further stated that, unlike earlier studies, all women included in their study had been diagnosed and were undergoing treatment.

Pop and Vulsma (2005) state that because the fetus does not produce thyroxine until mid gestation, and that brain development is very dependent on an adequate supply of thyroid hormones, it is essential that maternal iodine levels and thyroid hormones are adequate before conception and throughout pregnancy to ensure the future mental and motor skills of the developing fetus. Thyroxine requirements increase due to increased thyroid-binding globulin, greater plasma volume, and increased inactivation of T_4 and T_3 by the placenta (Bell & Hurel 2005). Close monitoring is therefore required and women should be kept on the lowest dose possible (Tan & Hurel 2001).

Labour and delivery are usually uneventful, although thyroid hormone levels should be assessed prior to term. Some studies state that women with hypothyroidism are unduly sensitive to opioids; even small doses may lead to unconsciousness or even death (Malseed et al 1995).

Monitoring for pre-eclampsia should be carried out as it is likely to develop in up to 40% of women and will be managed as per unit protocol. The midwife should be aware of these potential problems when delivering care, documenting findings and seeking medical assistance where necessary. Ultrasonography will be used to confirm the small for gestational age fetus and birth will be expedited according to unit protocols or guidelines.

Postpartum management

Postnatal care should be provided as for all women. Breast-feeding should be encouraged while undergoing treatment for hypothyroidism. Thyroid hormone replacement, when provided in proper dosage level, crosses into breast milk in only minute quantities, and has no adverse effect on the baby. The period following birth is one where thyroid levels can fluctuate, so frequent blood testing every 3 months is recommended.

Postpartum thyroiditis

This condition, which tends to occur within 1–3 months of birth, may produce antibodies which damage thyroid tissue, thereby releasing thyroid hormone passively into the bloodstream and producing hyperthyroidism. During the recovery phase, thyroid levels may fall, producing either temporary or permanent hypothyroid disease, requiring long-term thyroid replacement therapy. This condition is fairly common, occurring in 8–10% of all women after pregnancy, and women at risk include those with a previous history of postpartum thyroiditis or those who can be shown to have thyroid antibodies in their blood but are not taking levothyroxine (thyroxine) (Becks & Burrow 2000).

Congenital hypothyroidism

Screening in the UK detects congenital hypothyroidism in 1:4000 neonates (Shepherd et al 2006). Congenital hypothyroidism (Box 10.3) occurs when the thyroid gland fails to develop or function properly. In 80–85% of cases, the thyroid gland is absent, abnormally located, or severely reduced in size (hypoplastic). In the remaining cases, a normal-sized or enlarged thyroid gland is present, but production of thyroid hormones is decreased or absent (Israel et al 2006). Infants may present with some or all of the signs of congenital hypothyroidism (Table 10.5).

Box 10.3 Congenital hypothyroidism

If untreated, congenital hypothyroidism can lead to mental retardation and abnormal growth (Shepherd et al 2004). Infants with severe degrees of congenital hypothyroidism are seldom seen in the UK nowadays, as all infants are screened using the dry spot blood test at 4–6 days following birth. This screening aims to identify neonates with a high risk of the disorder. The diagnosis is then confirmed by further blood tests and clinical examination, and treatment with levothyroxine (thyroxine) established within 21 days to ensure normal development. The infant will be closely monitored by a paediatric endocrinologist, although as the child grows, hospital visits will be less frequent. Almost all children who are diagnosed and treated from an early age will develop normally.

Table 10.5   Signs of congenital hypothyroidism

- Large fontanelles
- Low hairline
- Protruding tongue
- Difficulty in maintaining thermoregulation
- Protruding umbilicus
- Growth failure
- Difficulty in feeding
- Constipation
- Short, thick neck
- Short arms and legs
- Broad hands with short fingers

REFERENCES

Becks G P, Burrow G N 2000 Thyroid disorders and pregnancy. Thyroid Foundation of Canada, London, Ontario

Bell R, Hurel S 2005 Hypothyroidism: A guide to clinical practice. Practice Nursing 16(7):329–333

British National Formulary (BNF) 2005 British National Formulary, No 50. British Medical Association and the Royal Pharmaceutical Society of Great Britain, London

de Swiet M, Chamberlain G, Bennet P 2002 Basic science in obstetrics and gynaecology: A textbook for MRCOG, Part 1, 3rd edn. Churchill Livingstone, Edinburgh

Dibbs C 2001 Nursing practice, hospital and home. In: Alexander M F, Fawcett J N, Runcimann P J (eds) The adult, 2nd edn. Churchill Livingstone, Edinburgh

Fordyce F 2002 Healthy rocks and wildlife farming. Planet Earth. Natural Environment Research Council, Swindon

Heuston W J 2001 Treatment of hypothyroidism. American Family Physician 64(10):1717–1724

Israel J, Parsons E P, Bradley D M 2006 Advances in newborn blood screening. British Journal of Midwifery 14(12):702–705

Jordan S 2002 Pharmacology for midwives. Palgrave, Houndmills

Kettyle W M, Arky R A 1998 Endocrine pathophysiology. Lippincott-Raven, Philadelphia

Kumar P, Clark M 2002 Clinical medicine, 5th edn. WB Saunders, Edinburgh

Lazarus J 2004 Screening for thyroid disease in pregnancy and the postpartum. Dept. of Medicine, University of Wales College of Medicine, Cardiff. Endocrine Nurses Training Course Wills Hall, Stoke Bishop, Bristol BS9 1AE

Lazarus J H, Premawardhana L D K E 2005 Best practice, No 184. Screening for thyroid disease in pregnancy. Journal of Clinical Pathology 58:449–452

Malseed R T, Goldstein F J, Balcon N 1995 Pharmacology: drug therapy and nursing considerations, 4th edn. Lippincott, Philadelphia.

Marieb E N, Hoehn K 2007 Human anatomy and physiology, 7th edn. San Francisco, Pearson Education

Marshall W 1999 Disorders of thyroid functioning. Practice Nursing 10(5):29–32

Martini F H 2005 Anatomy and physiology. Pearson Education, San Francisco

Perry M 2003 Hypothyroidism: More common in women. Practice Nursing 14(7):316–319

Pop V, Vulsma T 2005 Maternal hypothyroxinaemia during (early) gestation. Lancet 365(9471):1604–1607

Pop V, Baar A, Vulsma T 1999 Should all pregnant women be screened for hypothyroidism. Lancet 354:1224–1225

Schroeder B 2002 ACOG Practice bulletin on thyroid disease in pregnancy. American Family Physician 65(10):S1–S5

Shepherd A, Glenesk A, Niven C 2004 Evidence based approaches to neonatal screening. British Journal of Midwifery 12(12):762–766

Shepherd A, Glenesk A, Niven C, Mackenzie J 2006 Blood spot testing: Comparing techniques and automated devices. British Journal of Midwifery 14(2):96–99

Stables D, Rankin J 2005 Physiology in childbearing, 2nd edn. Elsevier, Edinburgh

Tan T, Hurel S 2001 A guide to common thyroid problems. Practice Nursing 12(5):190–193

Toft A 2004 Increased levothyroxine requirements in pregnancy – why, when, and how much? New England Journal of Medicine 351(3):292–294

Watkinson M 2003 Nursing patients with endocrine and metabolic disorders. In: Booker C, Nicol M (eds) Nursing adults: The practice of caring. Mosby, Edinburgh

Wolfberg A J, Lee-Parritz A, Peller A J, Lieberman E S 2005 Obstetric and neonatal outcomes associated with maternal hypothyroid disease. Journal of Maternal-Fetal and Neonatal Medicine 17(1):35–38

Chapter 11

Eating disorders

CHAPTER CONTENTS

INTRODUCTION

A well-balanced diet, full of all necessary nutrients, is essential to fetal growth and welfare. The fetus is considered to be a parasite removing from its mother's body all requirements whether she has sufficient herself or not. A deficit in certain nutrients at a crucial stage of fetal development may result in congenital abnormality or developmental problems. The role of folic acid in preventing a neural tube defect is an example of this.

At the first visit, the midwife should ask about the woman's diet and consider whether she is under- or overweight. This observation may give some indication of the woman's diet. Women who are above or below the healthy range of body weight are more at risk during pregnancy as are their babies. This section will consider the very sensitive issue of obesity and other eating disorders (Ratnaike 2007).

OBESITY

Obesity is on the increase in many parts of the developed world. In the UK, it is estimated that 32% of women between 35–64 years of age have a body mass index (BMI) of $25-30\,kg/m^2$ and 21% a BMI $>30\,kg/m^2$. Obesity in pregnant women carries an increased risk of maternal and fetal morbidity and mortality and in the most recent Confidential Enquiries into Maternal and Child

Health Report, 35% of the women who died were obese (Lewis & Drife 2004). Obesity was a major factor in these deaths.

Relevant physiology

Obesity is a chronic condition in which there is an excess amount of body fat. Some body fat is required by the body in which to store energy, insulate the body against a cold environment and to cover and protect the bones and organs of the body. Normal body fat is generally expressed as a percentage of body mass and should be between 25–30% in women (18–23% in men) and individuals with a higher percentage are considered obese.

Body weight depends in part on the genetic make-up of the individual and in part on the balance between food intake and energy expenditure of the body. Food intake is the only source of energy for performing all the biological reactions on which body function relies. These metabolic processes occur in all the cells of the body; chemical substances are taken into the cell where under the guidance of deoxyribonucleic acid (DNA) and the influence of enzymes, new products are formed.

Anabolism is the process by which chemical reactions combine to form more complex molecules, such as proteins, e.g. hormones, and glycogen for storage in the liver (see Ch. 9). Catabolism is the opposite process. Complex molecules are broken down into simple substances to enable these substances to be readily available to body cells. A by-product of catabolism is the release of energy which is required to fuel many anabolic reactions. The molecule that participates in most energy exchanges in body cells is adenosine triphosphate (ATP) which is utilized and rebuilt constantly. Heat is another vital by-product of metabolism ensuring that the human body temperature is largely independent of external temperature (Box 11.1)

A stable body weight is dependent on a balance between food intake and energy output. Food intake is measured in calories. Should an individual's calorific intake exceed the number of calories used in body functioning, the excess calories are stored in the body for times when food is scarce. In the developed world, this rarely

---

Box 11.1 Heat loss in the neonate

One of the functions of fat is to insulate the body against the cold. The newborn infant however has an added physiological aid to this process: brown fat. Brown fat is so named because it contains a higher number of blood vessels than normal fat. In the newborn infant, brown fat is stored in various places throughout the body and can be utilized to aid heat production at times of cold stress. This process, non-shivering thermogenesis, allows the mobilization of fatty acids and glycerol to produce heat at times when the infant is exposed to the cold environment. The normal term infant has sufficient brown fat to meet minimum heat needs for 2–4 days after birth. The pre-term infant or the neonate with intrauterine growth restriction will however have a deficit of both normal subcutaneous fat and brown fat and is thus more at risk of hypothermia.

---

happens. Over time, an individual who constantly takes in too many calories will increase in weight to a greater or lesser extent, depending on the degree of overeating.

Other factors involved are thought to be eating a diet high in simple carbohydrates and the frequency of eating. Simple carbohydrates are absorbed rapidly and cause large swings in blood sugar levels. This results in cravings for food which is often taken as snacks (Box 11.2). Eating large meals infrequently also does this, especially if the meals taken are also largely composed of easily digested foodstuffs.

Box 11.2 Glycaemic index

Glycaemic index (GI) is a ranking system for carbohydrates based on their effect on blood glucose levels after digestion. Carbohydrates that break down rapidly after ingestion cause blood glucose levels to rise rapidly; those that take longer to digest result in a slower rise and consequently a slower fall. Rapidly digested carbohydrates are given a high GI. For a healthy and satisfying diet therefore, basing meals on low GI foods prevents rapid rises and falls in blood sugars, which are also associated with cravings for fast foods and snacks with high sugar content.

Psychological factors play a large part in obesity; emotions influence eating habits. Many people eat excessively in response to emotions, such as boredom, sadness, stress or anger. Racial factors play a part with African-American women and Hispanic women putting on weight earlier in life than Caucasian women. The female hormone oestrogen is also thought to have some influence on weight gain – when on the contraceptive pill, during pregnancy and during the menopause. Diseases such as hypothyroidism, polycystic ovaries and Cushing's syndrome are also contributors to obesity.

Many of the above factors however are additionally linked to an individual's metabolic rate. Metabolic rate is the rate at which the body breaks down nutrients to liberate energy. Many factors affect metabolic rate and these may significantly influence whether or not an individual gains weight.

- *Exercise*: during strenuous exercise, the metabolic rate may increase 15-fold
- *Stress*: noradrenaline increases the metabolic rate
- *Hormones*: thyroid hormones, testosterone and human growth hormone all increase the metabolic rate
- *Body temperature*: increasing temperature as in fever, results in increasing metabolic rate
- *Ingestion of food* raises the metabolic rate by 10–20% and is particularly related to the intake of protein
- *Age*: the metabolic rate of a child is much greater than an adult. An elderly individual will have a decreased metabolic rate. Much of this is related to growth and activity
- *Other factors*: increased metabolic rate is found in pregnancy and lactation; decreased metabolic rate with malnutrition (including dieting), living in tropical regions and during sleep.

Obesity is more than a cosmetic consideration – it carries a greatly increased risk of premature death and disease processes. Briefly these are mentioned below.

Hypertension

Raised blood pressure is common among obese adults. The cardiovascular system has to increase cardiac output to transport blood around the extra body mass. This can only continue for a limited time without increasing blood pressure, and this rises especially if there are additional factors such as arteriosclerosis present. Related to all these changes, and linked also to diet and genetics, high cholesterol levels may cause further disease processes.

Insulin resistance

Insulin is required to transport glucose into body cells (see Ch. 9) for use as an energy source to fuel chemical reactions. Excess glucose in blood damages body structures and organs. Fat cells are resistant to insulin and the pancreas responds by increasing the amount of insulin produced. While the pancreas can produce enough insulin to overcome this resistance, blood glucose levels remain normal. This condition of normal blood glucose levels with high blood insulin levels can persist for years. Once the pancreas can no longer maintain this level of production, blood glucose levels begin to rise, and the individual develops type 2 diabetes.

Other conditions

The above changes will increase the risks of cardiovascular accident (stroke) and heart attacks among obese individuals. Also, some cancers appear to be related to obesity. Due to the high levels of fats circulating in the bloodstream, gallstones are also more prevalent (see Ch. 12).

Diagnosis

Although the definition of obesity is based on the proportion of fat in the body, it is extremely difficult to accurately measure this. Diagnosis is therefore commonly based on body mass index (BMI).

BMI is a mathematical formula that accounts for an individual's weight and height. The BMI equals that person's weight in kilograms (kg) divided by height in metres squared (m^2).

$$BMI = kg/m^2$$

There is some debate about the value of the BMI as a tool for identifying a 'healthy' versus an 'unhealthy' range. It also gives no indication of the percentage of fat in the body. However, it is a useful guideline for adults. Care must be taken if used for children, some athletes and pregnant women. A 'healthy' weight is usually identified by a BMI between 19 and 25 in healthy adults (Tables 11.1, 11.2). Obesity is usually considered to be a BMI >30.

Table 11.1 Calculation of BMI

BMI (kg/m^2)	19	20	21	22	23	24	25	26	27	28	29	30	35	40
Height (in)							Weight (lbs)							
58	91	96	100	105	110	115	119	124	129	134	138	143	167	191
59	94	99	104	109	114	119	124	128	133	138	143	148	173	198
60	97	102	107	112	118	123	128	133	138	143	148	153	179	204
61	100	106	111	116	122	127	132	137	143	148	153	158	185	211
62	104	109	115	120	126	131	136	142	147	153	158	164	191	218
63	107	113	118	124	130	135	141	146	152	158	163	169	197	225
64	110	116	122	128	134	140	145	151	157	163	169	174	204	232
65	114	120	126	132	138	144	150	156	162	168	174	180	210	240
66	118	124	130	136	142	148	155	161	167	173	179	186	216	247
67	121	127	134	140	146	153	159	166	172	178	185	191	223	255
68	125	131	138	144	151	158	164	171	177	184	190	197	230	262
69	128	135	142	149	155	162	169	176	182	189	196	203	236	270
70	132	139	146	153	160	167	174	181	188	195	202	207	243	278
71	136	143	150	157	165	172	179	186	193	200	208	215	250	286
72	140	147	154	162	169	177	184	191	199	206	213	221	258	294
73	144	151	159	166	174	182	189	197	204	212	219	227	265	302
74	148	155	163	171	179	186	194	202	210	218	225	233	272	311
75	152	160	168	176	184	192	200	208	216	224	232	240	279	319
76	156	164	172	180	189	197	205	213	221	230	238	246	287	328

Table 11.2 Relationship between BMI and obesity

BMI	Category	Waist ≤40 in (men) or ≤35 in (women)	Waist >40 in (men) or >35 in (women)
<18.5	Underweight	N/A	N/A
18.5–24.9	Normal	N/A	N/A
25.0–29.9	Overweight	Increased risk	High risk
30.0–34.9	Obese	High risk	Very high risk
35.0–39.9	Obese	Very high risk	Very high risk
≥40	Extremely obese	Extremely high risk	Extremely high risk

Treatment

Dieting is not necessarily the answer to overweight or obesity (NICE 2006). Dealing with this problem involves a detailed look at lifestyle, stress, external influences and eating patterns. Dieting alone often leads to a return to a pre-diet weight within a few years. Changing one's lifestyle by dealing with stress, modifying the diet, increasing exercise and identifying achievable steady weight loss will have a significant effect both on obesity and the risks associated with them.

OBESITY IN PREGNANCY AND CHILDBIRTH

During pregnancy and childbirth, metabolism is adjusted under the influence of the endocrine glands to ensure that adequate nutrients are available to support the growth and development of the fetus and to provide energy reserves for the demands of the childbearing process.

Pregnancy is a time of increased anabolism in which food intake and appetite are increased, activity is decreased and energy reserves of approximately 30 000 kcal are established (Blackburn 2002). The increase in anabolism is greatest in the first and second trimesters of pregnancy and maternal weight increases largely due to fat deposition. During the third trimester of pregnancy, weight gain is primarily due to the growing fetus and placenta despite maternal fat stores being utilized.

Pregnancy complicated by obesity

Pregnancy is associated with increased demands on the cardiovascular system as a result of the presence of the fetoplacental unit and the increase in size of the uterus, breasts, etc. Obesity adds an additional demand on this process. For every additional 100 g of fat present in the body, cardiac output has to increase by 30–50 mL/min (Yu et al 2006). This is also accompanied by an increase in blood volume. If the increases in load are considerable, the heart muscle may hypertrophy, which will disrupt the normal functioning of the heart.

Additionally, hypertension may already be present in the obese woman before pregnancy. Pre-eclampsia has been found to present in over 10% of obese pregnant women and 12% of morbidly obese women, compared with 4.8% in a comparable normal weight population (Kabiru & Raynor 2004). A systematic review of BMI and the risk of pre-eclampsia showed that the risk of pre-eclampsia typically doubled with each $5–7 \text{kg/m}^2$ (O'Brien et al 2003). The risk of thromboembolism doubles in obese women (Sebire et al 2001) and gestational diabetes develops in three times more obese women than in those with a normal BMI (Weiss et al 2004).

Infertility and spontaneous abortion is increased in obese women and obstetric complications are an issue for the multidisciplinary team. Monitoring of the mother and the fetus is difficult in the obese woman. Anaesthetic risks are increased. Shoulder dystocia, instrumental delivery and caesarean section rates are all increased in the obese women (Yu et al 2006). However, these may be caused in part by the defensive care given to the woman in labour – labouring and giving birth on a bed will restrict pelvic diameters (Box 11.3).

In the puerperium, infection rates are increased. Postpartum haemorrhage rises with increasing BMI and is 30% more likely in women with moderately raised BMI and 70% more likely in women with a greatly increased BMI (Sebire et al 2001).

Box 11.3 Pelvic diameters

Women who are encouraged to adopt their own most comfortable position for labour and birth seldom lie in a bed. The involvement of the medical profession has led to the adoption of the semi-recumbent position for birth, especially in women who require extra monitoring during labour. However, this position restricts the ability of the pelvis to increase its diameters as the fetus moves through the birth canal.

In women who are at particular risk of birthing a baby above average in weight, there is a considerable advantage to encouraging the woman to adopt an upright position. This will allow gravity to aid descent and to encourage the fetus to adapt to the available space within the pelvic cavity. The midwife can encourage movement and mobility to some degree with the majority of women despite the need for closer monitoring in those at risk and thus promote a spontaneous vaginal birth.

Obesity in the pregnant women increases fetal mortality and morbidity. Identification of congenital abnormality is difficult and studies are ambivalent about the incidence of congenital abnormalities in obese women. However, macrosomia has been found to be more common (Cedergren 2004). This appears to be related to the presence of insulin resistance in the mother with high blood glucose and/or insulin resulting in hyperinsulinaemia in the fetus (see Ch. 9). Perinatal mortality rate is also increased in the fetus of an obese woman. There is a two-fold increase in both stillbirth and neonatal death (Kristensen et al 2005). No clear explanation has been found for these deaths.

Long-term outcomes are also poor for infants of obese women. Large for gestational age neonates appear to be at greatly increased risk of obesity in adult life (Baird et al 2005).

Management of obesity in pregnancy and childbirth

Ideally, all women should be seen before pregnancy for preconception advice. As the aim of this service is to achieve optimal health before conception, this would be particularly helpful in the case of a woman with a weight problem. Discussing with the woman and her partner the increased risks both to herself and to her baby, may encourage the woman to make lifestyle changes before becoming pregnant. Examination before pregnancy will also enable the midwife to identify baseline observations of blood pressure and urinalysis, which will be useful in gauging the changes during pregnancy.

Early in pregnancy, the midwife will be able to sensitively bring up the issue of weight and offer referral to a dietician. It is not advisable to diet during pregnancy as vital nutrients may be missing from the diet; however a sensible healthy eating pattern will be discussed and the woman encouraged to put on minimal weight during the pregnancy (King 2006). Careful observations of blood pressure and urinalysis will be undertaken at all antenatal visits and an ongoing risk assessment for thromboembolic complications considered.

Labour and birth should be encouraged in an obstetric unit because of the difficulties in identification of presentation and position of the fetus and of monitoring the fetus during labour. Additionally, as discussed above, there are increased risks to both mother and baby during the birthing process. Birth under the care of the multidisciplinary team will allow prompt treatment if there are difficulties with the birth or postnatally. However, the midwife should give the woman every opportunity to remain active during labour and birth and discourage birth in any position that restricts the diameters of the pelvis as the fetus may be above average in weight.

Postnatally, the midwife should be alert for signs of deep venous thrombosis or infection. The mother should be advised to keep mobile and to care for her baby. Extra help may be required with breast-feeding – positioning may need to be adjusted to enable the baby to attach correctly to the breast. Again the midwife can take every opportunity to educate the mother regarding diet and exercise (Bainbridge 2006) and can introduce the woman to supportive services.

ANOREXIA AND BULIMIA

The Confidential Enquiry into Maternal Deaths 2000–2002 reported that severe mental illness caused or contributed to 12% of maternal deaths, 10% of which were due to suicide (Lewis & Drife 2004). Eating disorders are a symptom of mental illness and are increasing in prevalence (Martos-Ordonez 2005) and pregnancy is a time when women suffering from these conditions are likely to become more anxious about their body image. Midwives must therefore be vigilant for indications of one of the eating disorders and be aware of the necessary pathways for managing the condition.

Anorexia nervosa and bulimia nervosa affect many women of childbearing age. These eating disorders were found to be at least five times more prevalent in the female population than the male with an overall incidence in females of $\leqslant 0.5\%$ in a recent large study in Sweden (Lindberg & Hjern 2003). These illnesses are characterized by severe disturbances in eating behaviour, such as severe restriction of food intake or binge eating as well as extreme anxiety about body weight or body shape. Eating disorders such as these are an expression of deep psychological and emotional problems in which sufferers make use of food in diverse ways in an effort to manage their distress.

Anorexia nervosa is a condition in which the individual is found to have a 15% reduction in weight below the normal range with amenorrhoea of at least 3 months' duration. In anorexia, the appetite is initially normal but as the disease progresses, appetite decreases. The individual with anorexia may display two distinct eating behaviours: a restrictive form, in which the types and amounts of foods are severely limited, and binge eating or purging, in which women induce vomiting after eating or use purging methods such as laxatives, diuretics or enemas. These behaviours result in a deterioration in health, as well as severe weight loss. Yet despite this weight loss and the resulting pathologically thin body, the woman still sees herself as fat. Depression and obsessive compulsive behaviour frequently occur alongside anorexia (James 2001).

Bulimia nervosa is defined as two or more episodes of binge eating every week for at least 3 weeks followed by vomiting or purging through the use of laxatives or diuretics (James 2001). This cycle is frequently interspersed with fasting or exercise. Bulimia is not necessarily associated with weight loss – the woman may be of normal weight or even slightly overweight. Bulimia is more common than anorexia, with up to 20% of women experiencing bulimia or bulimia-like symptoms at some time during their life time (James 2001).

Pregnancy is rare in women who are considerably underweight, as they commonly suffer amenorrhoea. In those women who do achieve a pregnancy, there is an increase in complications such as pre-eclampsia and hypertension, breech presentation and caesarean section (Martos-Ordonez 2005). Hyperemesis is also seen more frequently. For the fetus, spontaneous abortion, intrauterine death, fetal distress, jaundice, poor weight gain and pre-term birth are all more common.

Pregnancy in women with an eating disorder often presents the individual with a dilemma. These women fear becoming fat during pregnancy. They fear a loss of control as they experience an increased appetite, an enlarging abdomen and larger breasts (James 2001). Personal issues which have been suppressed may surface and pose challenges to the pregnant woman. Diagnosis of pregnancy may be delayed as irregularities in menstruation are commonplace. The difficulty for those caring for women with eating disorders is to ensure that an adequate well-balanced diet is being taken at a time when the fetus is most at risk. However, many individuals will not disclose their illness as they wish to avoid treatment that may result in weight gain (Wolfe 2005).

Caring for a woman with an eating disorder is the responsibility of the multidisciplinary team. This is a pregnancy that is at greater risk than in women of normal weight and diet and thus the midwife must refer her with consent to the appropriate medical practitioner. The use of cognitive behavioural therapy may be a component of this care (James 2001) and the use of relaxation techniques may enable the woman to control her guilt about eating or weight gain. Medications are also useful but these cross the placenta and a careful evaluation of the risks and benefits of therapy will be considered by the multidisciplinary team.

While caring for the woman, the midwife may find that by focussing the woman's attention on the fetus, eating patterns improve. A discussion of the essential components of a well-balanced diet will be required as many woman do not have a good understanding of this. However, the early postnatal period is a peak time for relapse or deterioration of the eating disorder and the midwife should refer promptly to the psychiatric team (Morrill & Nickols-Richardson 2001). The midwife should also be alert for other psychiatric disorders, such as anxiety and depression, as these are more common in women with eating disorders.

REFERENCES

Bainbridge 2006 Lingering pregnancy fat puts women in danger. British Journal of Midwifery 14(11):644

Baird J, Fisher D, Lucas P, Kleijnen J, Robert H, Lae C 2005 Being too big or growing fast: systematic review of size in infancy and later obesity. British Medical Journal 331:929

Blackburn S 2002 Maternal, fetal and neonatal physiology: A clinical perspective, 2nd edn. WB Saunders, Philadelphia

Cedergren MI 2004 Maternal morbid obesity and the risk of adverse pregnancy outcome. Obstetrics and Gynecology 103: 219–224

Lewis G, Drife J (eds) 2004 Why Mothers Die 2000–2002. The sixth report of the Confidential Enquires into Maternal Deaths in the United Kingdom. RCOG, London

James DC 2001 Eating disorders, fertility and pregnancy: Relationships and complications. Journal of Perinatal & Neonatal Nursing 15(2):36–48

Kabiru W, Raynor B D 2004 Obstetric outcomes associated with increase in BMI category during pregnancy. American Journal of Obstetrics and Gynecology 191:928–932

King J C 2006 Maternal obesity, metabolism and pregnancy outcomes. Annual Review of Nutrition 26:271–291

Kristensen J, Vestergaard M, Wisborg K, Kesmodel U, Secher N J 2005 Pre-pregnancy weight and the risk of stillbirth and neonatal death. British Journal of Obstetrics and Gynaecology 112:403–408

Lindberg L, Hjern A 2003 Risk factors for anorexia nervosa: A national cohort study. International Journal of Eating Disorders 34:397–408

Martos-Ordonez C 2005 Pregnancy in women with eating disorders: a review. British Journal of Midwifery 13(7):446–448

Morrill E S, Nickols-Richardson H M 2001 Bulimia during pregnancy: a review. Journal of the American Dietetics Association 101(4):448–454

National Institute for Clinical Excellence 2006 Obesity: the prevention, identification, assessment and management of overweight and obesity in adults and children. Clinical Guideline 43. NICE, London

O'Brien T E, Ray J G, Chan W S 2003 Maternal body mass index and the risk of pre-eclampsia: A systematic review. Epidemiology 14:368–374

Ratnaike D 2007 Eating disorders: Shame and secrecy. RCM Midwives Journal 10(4):156

Sebire N J, Jolly M, Harris J P, Wadsworth J, Jaffe M, Beard R W et al 2001 Maternal obesity and pregnancy outcome: a study of 287,213 pregnancies in London. International Journal of Obesity Related Metabolic Disorders 25:1175–1182

Weiss J L, Malone F D, Emig D et al 2004 Obesity, obstetric complications and caesarean delivery rate – a population based screening study. American Journal of Obstetrics and Gynecology 190:1091–1097

Wolfe B E 2005 Reproductive health in women with eating disorders. Journal of Obstetric, Gynecological and Neonatal Nursing (34)2:255–263

Yu C K H, Teoh T G, Robinson S 2006 Obesity in pregnancy. British Journal of Obstetrics and Gynaecology 113:1117–1125

Chapter 12

Disorders of the gastrointestinal system

INTRODUCTION

During the childbearing process, the gastrointestinal (GI) system is affected both by the hormones of pregnancy and by its displacement by the growing fetus. It is not uncommon therefore for the pregnant woman to complain of, e.g. abdominal discomfort and changes to bowel habits. It is also as likely during pregnancy as at any other time of the woman's life that she develops problems related to the GI tract, such as appendicitis or cholecystitis. The midwife must therefore be vigilant to the possible causes – the differential diagnoses – of both pregnancy and non-pregnancy related conditions.

This chapter looks both at medical conditions related to the gastrointestinal system that may occur at any time in an individual's life and at those unique to pregnancy and childbirth.

RELEVANT ANATOMY AND PHYSIOLOGY OF THE GASTROINTESTINAL TRACT

Relatively common conditions experienced by the pregnant woman relate principally to the small and large intestines of the GI tract. These include inflammatory bowel disease and irritable bowel syndrome. Crohn's disease, one of the inflammatory conditions, can affect the entire length of the GI tract but in the early stages of the disease tends to affect the intestines. This section will therefore discuss this area of the GI tract only.

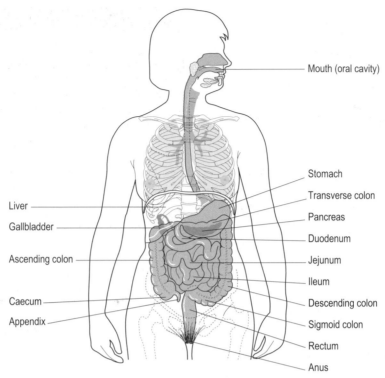

Figure 12.1   The gastrointestinal tract.

The small intestine extends from the distal sphincter of the stomach to the ileocaecal sphincter at the junction with the large intestine (Fig. 12.1). The small intestine is divided into the duodenum, jejunum and ileum, which are each highly adapted to digestion and absorption. The walls of the small intestine are folded (Fig. 12.2) to produce a large surface area for these processes. Glands secrete mucus and fluids, and the brush border provides enzymes to reduce proteins, carbohydrates and fats to their basic components for ease of absorption.

The large intestine, the caecum, colon, rectum and anal canal, extends from the ileocaecal sphincter to the anus. This section of the gastrointestinal tract is responsible for absorption of water, electrolytes and vitamins, thus concentrating the faeces to prevent loss of fluid from the body. Some final chemical digestion is performed by resident bacteria. Waste products in the form of faeces are then eliminated from the body by defecation, through the anus.

INFLAMMATORY BOWEL DISEASE

Inflammatory bowel disease (IBD) is on the increase in the developed world and thus an increasing number of women are becoming pregnant with this disorder. Inflammatory bowel disease includes the two conditions: ulcerative colitis and Crohn's disease.

The cause of this disease is unknown. There appears to be a genetic predisposition to the condition but it is thought to be an autoimmune disease – the patient's own immune system attacks the intestine causing inflammation. Both conditions commonly first occur in young people in their teens to 20s.

Ulcerative colitis is a disorder of the colon and rectum in which there is severe inflammation and oedema of the intestinal mucosa. Ulceration develops and the individual suffers from diarrhoea, urgency and abdominal pain. Ulcerative colitis varies in intensity and severity between individuals. The more severe forms result in malaise,

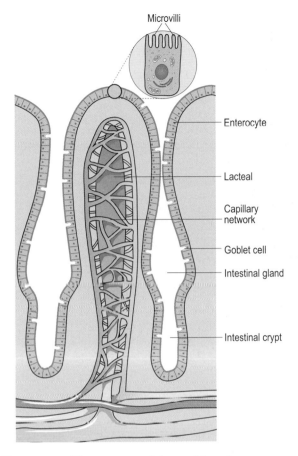

Microvilli

Enterocyte

Lacteal

Capillary network

Goblet cell

Intestinal gland

Intestinal crypt

Figure 12.2   Microstructure of the small intestine.

Box 12.1 Ileostomy/colostomy

An ileostomy is a stoma, a surgically created opening, which has been formed by bringing the end of the ileum out onto the surface of the skin. A colostomy is created from a portion of the colon. Intestinal waste products thus pass out of the body through the stoma and are collected in an external bag stuck to the abdominal surface. Ileostomy/colostomy is necessary where disease or injury has damaged the intestines preventing them from functioning adequately. The diseased portion of the intestine is removed and the stoma formed as an alternative. Patients with either Crohn's disease or ulcerative colitis may require this operation.

Dietary adjustments may be required after having an ileostomy or colostomy. High fibre foods may be hard to digest and cause discomfort when passing through the stoma. Foods that produce an increase in flatus also have to be avoided. Overall however, patients who require a stoma for IBD typically find that they can eat a more normal diet and are comparatively free from symptoms after this type of surgery.

fatigue and weight loss. Complications of the condition include anaemia, tachycardia, fever and dehydration.

Crohn's disease can affect any part of the gastrointestinal tract and is characterized by inflammation and ulceration of the entire depth of the wall of the intestine. Commonly, it affects the small intestine preventing adequate absorption of nutrients. Typically, the individual suffers from acute episodes of illness with long periods of mild and intermittent symptoms. During the acute stage, the individual suffers severe inflammatory symptoms of cramping pain, diarrhoea, flatulence, nausea and fever.

Treatment of both conditions can be medical or surgical. Medical treatment involves the use of anti-inflammatory and immunosuppressant drugs and steroids. Surgery includes removal of the affected part of the intestine. This may cure

ulcerative colitis as once removed it does not recur. In Crohn's disease however, surgery will only be undertaken if there is no other possible treatment, as there is a high incidence of recurrence. Generally surgery involves removal of the affected area and an anastomosis of the two healthy ends although a colostomy/ileostomy may be required (Box 12.1).

Both of these conditions can cause problems outside the gastrointestinal tract such as skin rashes, arthritis and inflammation of the eyes. There is an increased risk of gastrointestinal cancer. Both of these diseases are characterized by remissions and exacerbations. Inflammatory bowel disease can be very disruptive to the lives of the individuals who suffer from it. It affects the ability of the individuals to eat, participate in social and work activities and can have a major effect on the individual's character.

INFLAMMATORY BOWEL DISEASE AND CHILDBIRTH

The peak onset of inflammatory bowel disease is between 20 and 40 years of age and thus the impact of the disease on pregnancy is an important clinical issue. Generally, both diseases are thought to follow a similar course that existed before conception, i.e. if in remission, this will continue through pregnancy, while active disease is likely to complicate pregnancy leading to increased maternal and fetal morbidity (Bush et al 2004). The risk of a relapse during pregnancy is considered to be 33%, which is no higher than in those not pregnant (www. crohn's.org.uk). A relapse is more likely during the first trimester of pregnancy and postnatally. Those individuals who have an ileostomy may find some dysfunction in the later stages of pregnancy when the growing fetus displaces the intestines.

Drugs used in the treatment of IBD are relatively safe for use in pregnancy – certainly the risks of the disease are higher than the risks from the medicines used to keep the condition in remission (Langarragard et al 2007). However, some studies have shown an increase in congenital abnormalities (Alstead & Nelson-Piercy 2003).

Supplementation with folic acid will be advised, as this vital substance for fetal development may not be adequately absorbed by the damaged gut.

Breast-feeding is not contraindicated either by the medication or from the effects of the disease process on the mother. The risk to the neonate of inheriting IBD is thought to be 8–9% (www. crohn's.org.uk).

IRRITABLE BOWEL SYNDROME

Irritable bowel syndrome (IBS) is a common bowel disorder in which the patient complains of abdominal pain and a change in bowel habit. It is the commonest reason for a consultation with the gastroenterologist. The condition may occur following an acute infectious illness, however in the majority of cases no cause is found. On examination, there are no apparent structural abnormalities and the condition does not disturb sleep. Symptoms commonly commence in young adulthood.

Factors that appear to be involved in this condition are:

- A genetic predisposition
- An increased sensitivity to noxious stimuli in the gut

- A previous episode of enteritis
- Food allergies and sensitivities
- Bacterial overgrowth in the intestines
- Stress
- Hormones, particularly those related to the female reproductive cycle.

Treatment is to examine the diet and consider which if any foods exacerbate the symptoms. Some patients find that cutting out dairy products, red meat, fats, coffee and artificial sweeteners substantially reduces the symptoms of IBS. Pharmacological treatment is based on symptom relief (Bruno 2004).

The effect of pregnancy on IBS varies considerably between individuals. Many women find that the abdominal pain and bowel problems worsen during menstruation and also during pregnancy. Others find that IBS completely disappears during pregnancy. IBS has no effect on the pregnancy however, as there has never been any evidence that the absorption of nutrients is affected in IBS.

APPENDICITIS

Appendicitis can occur in pregnancy as at any other stage of a woman's life and commonly at an advanced stage (Somani et al 2003). This may be because diagnosis is more difficult.

Appendicitis is an inflammation of the appendix, a largely redundant structure situated at the junction of the small and large intestine. Typically the patient complains of pain which starts around the umbilicus before localizing to the right iliac fossa. This is usually associated with loss of appetite and fever. Nausea and vomiting may also be present. Diagnosis is based on history and physical examination. Gentle palpation in the right iliac fossa will identify firm to rigid abdominal muscles with localized soreness if asked to cough. Rectal examination will reveal right-sided tenderness.

Peritonitis is a common complication if diagnosis and treatment are delayed. Intravenous antibiotics will be commenced and the patient starved until surgery can be arranged. Recovery is usually uneventful.

MEDICAL CONDITIONS RELATED TO THE ACCESSORY ORGANS OF DIGESTION

The accessory organs of digestion include the liver, pancreas and gallbladder. Diabetes mellitus is a condition in which the islets of Langerhans in the pancreas dysfunction. This condition however is described in Chapter 9, as these structures have an endocrine function. Obstetric cholestasis, involving the liver and gallbladder is a condition of pregnancy that is associated with a high fetal mortality rate.

Obstetric cholestasis

Intrahepatic cholestasis of pregnancy is the most common disorder of the liver peculiar to pregnancy and one that is still poorly recognized by both midwives and medical practitioners. The symptoms of the condition are relatively mild but become more distressing with increasing gestation. The effect can be devastating to both mother and baby. Thus, the midwife must be aware of its distinguishing features in order to advise the mother appropriately.

Relevant anatomy and physiology

The structures involved in obstetric cholestasis are the liver and the gallbladder (Fig. 12.3). Both of these structures are accessory organs of the gastrointestinal system and are involved in several vital processes.

The liver is the largest gland in the body, weighing approximately 1.5 kg in the adult. It is situated in the right hypochondriac region of the abdominal cavity, under the diaphragm, partially protected by the lower ribs. It is essential to life but can continue to function even when a large portion of its mass has been destroyed by illness or disease.

The liver is enclosed in a dense capsule of connective tissue and is divided into right and left lobes. The falciform ligament divides the lobes and attaches the organ to the lower aspect of the diaphragm. A second ligament, the ligamentum teres, also secures the liver in position and extends from the falciform ligament to the inner surface of the umbilicus. During fetal life, the ligamentum teres was in fact the umbilical vein running through the umbilical cord.

Microscopically, the liver is composed of a large number of hepatic lobules which are the functional

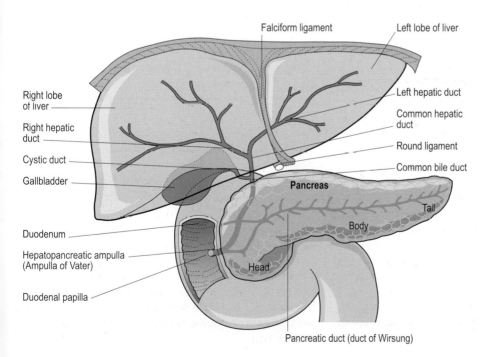

Falciform ligament — Left lobe of liver

Right lobe of liver

Right hepatic duct

Cystic duct

Gallbladder

Duodenum

Hepatopancreatic ampulla (Ampulla of Vater)

Duodenal papilla

Left hepatic duct

Common hepatic duct

Round ligament

Common bile duct

Pancreas

Tail

Body

Head

Pancreatic duct (duct of Wirsung)

Figure 12.3 Structure and relevant positions of liver and gallbladder.

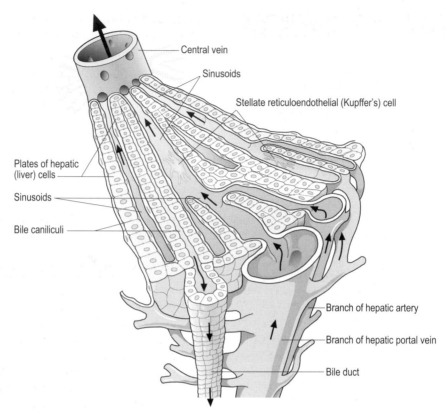

Figure 12.4   Microstructure of the liver.

units of the organ. Each lobule is composed of liver cells, hepatocytes, which are arranged in branching interconnected plates around a central vein (Fig. 12.4). Running between the hepatocytes are sinuses lined with specialized cells, reticuloendothelial (Kupffer's) cells. Around the circumference of the lobules are portal canals which carry a branch of the portal vein, hepatic artery and a small bile duct.

The liver receives blood from two sources. The hepatic artery brings oxygenated blood from the heart, while the hepatic portal vein brings deoxygenated blood directly from the gastrointestinal system. Branches of both these blood vessels enter the hepatic sinuses and thus hepatocytes can extract oxygen and nutrients for use by body cells, and some poisons which are detoxified in the liver. Additionally Kupffer's cells phagocytize microbes, foreign matter and damaged cells from the blood.

Bile is produced in the liver by the hepatocytes. Some 750–1000 mL of bile is produced every day and stored and concentrated in the gallbladder, which is situated beneath the liver (Fig. 12.3). This fluid is a viscous, alkaline, greenish yellow substance which contains water, bile salts, bile pigments, phospholipids, cholesterol and electrolytes. Bile is released intermittently in response to digestive hormones and is involved in excretion and in the breakdown of fats. Many of the components of bile are recycled by reabsorption into the blood in the ileum and returned to the liver by the enterohepatic circulation.

Bile salts are involved in emulsifying (breaking down) large molecules of fats into small droplets, which can then be more readily digested by pancreatic lipase. The principal bile pigment is bilirubin, which comes from the breakdown of red blood cells (Box 12.2). Fat soluble bilirubin is converted in the

Box 12.2 Jaundice

Jaundice is a symptom of a disease process. The condition describes a yellowing of the skin, conjunctiva of the eyes and the mucous membranes. Jaundice is caused by increased levels of unconjugated, fat soluble, bilirubin in the body. Bilirubin is a by-product of the breakdown of red blood cells. Haem, one of the components of red blood cells, is converted to bilirubin in the spleen, and then into a water soluble form in the liver and can then be excreted via bile in faeces. Jaundice will therefore be the result of a failure in some part of this process.

Haemolytic jaundice occurs when too many red blood cells are broken down and the body cannot cope with the amount of bilirubin requiring conversion to its water soluble form. A hepatic form occurs when the liver is not functioning correctly. Extrahepatic jaundice occurs when there is a problem with the removal of bile. Physiological jaundice in the newborn is the result of an inability of the immature liver to cope with the extra red blood cells that are being broken down after birth. This condition will resolve within a few days of birth but care must be taken to identify hyperbilirubi-naemia, which can lead to kernicterus.

liver to a water soluble form which is then excreted by the gastrointestinal system.

The liver therefore performs many vital functions, which include:

- Carbohydrate metabolism: The liver regulates blood glucose levels within very fine limits by converting glucose to glycogen in response to insulin, and glycogen back to glucose in response to glucagon

- Protein metabolism: In the liver, proteins are broken down and their waste products prepared for excretion. The liver then manufactures a variety of other proteins such as plasma proteins, albumin and clotting factors

- Fat metabolism: The liver is involved in the breakdown of fatty acids and the storage of triglycerides. The liver also manufactures lipoproteins and cholesterol

- Removal of drugs and hormones: The liver is responsible for detoxifying and excreting some drugs and poisons, as well as deactivating hormones no longer required in the body

- Storage: As well as glycogen, the liver is involved in the storage of vitamins A, B_{12}, D, E and K, and the minerals iron and copper. Iron is stored in the liver as ferritin

- Secretion: Bile is produced and stored in the gallbladder, as described above. Urea is formed in the liver from waste products such as ammonia and carbon dioxide and transported in the blood to the kidneys for excretion

- Activation of Vitamin D: The liver, skin and kidneys are all involved in activating vitamin D.

Relevant physiological changes in pregnancy

The liver is anatomically displaced by the uterus as pregnancy advances and some metabolic processes are altered. Fat and glycogen storage is largely unchanged but the production of plasma proteins, bilirubin, serum enzymes and serum lipids is altered in response to increased oestrogen and also as a result of haemodilution. Albumin levels decrease; alkaline phosphate, cholesterol, liver proteins and fibrinogen levels all increase. Thus, although liver function is not normally impaired during pregnancy, liver function tests mimic those of individuals with liver disease and results should be interpreted with caution.

Despite the increase in circulating blood volume during pregnancy, the liver receives little of this. As a result, the proportion of cardiac output that is delivered to the liver is decreased by one-third (Riely & Fallon 1999).

The gallbladder becomes hypotonic due to the action of progesterone on the muscle walls. As a result, it is able to increase the amount of bile stored and thus the rate of emptying decreases. Concentration of bile is thus affected, resulting in more dilute bile and a corresponding decrease in the ability to convert cholesterol to its soluble form. There is an increased tendency to form cholesterol-based gallstones during pregnancy, especially in the second and third trimesters (Blackburn 2002). These tend to remain symptomless, however (Murray 2003). Additionally, bile salts tend to be retained, which can lead to pruritus.

OBSTETRIC CHOLESTASIS

Incidence

Obstetric cholestasis is the most common disorder of liver function peculiar to pregnancy. The incidence of the condition varies considerably between cultures with an overall prevalence ranging from 1 in 200 to 0.5 in 1000 in the UK (Kenyon et al 2002). The condition is more common in women of advanced maternal age and in multiple pregnancies (Nichols 2005).

Pathophysiology

Obstetric cholestasis presents as pruritus of the extremities usually in the third trimester, with biochemical disturbances in liver enzymes. Jaundice may be present. This condition is not well understood. There would appear to be a genetic and/or hormonal cause as a similar condition can occur in women who use the contraceptive pill (Riely & Fallon 1999). Overproduction of oestrogen by the fetoplacental unit has been suggested as a cause. The condition occurs mainly in the third trimester when oestrogen levels are at their highest and resolves soon after birth. An alternative theory is that it is the result of a genetic predisposition which causes an increased sensitivity to oestrogen subsequently resulting in a metabolic defect in the hepatocytes. Whatever the aetiology of the disorder, the result is a disturbance in the enterohepatic circulation causing an accumulation of bile salts in the blood. This impedes the absorption of fat soluble vitamins, such as vitamin K, with corresponding coagulation defects. Additionally, the elevated levels of bile salts in the blood trigger the release of histamine causing the intense pruritus related to cholestasis.

Diagnosis

Alterations in normal liver function tests during pregnancy make diagnosis of liver dysfunction difficult. Serial liver function tests will show a steady increase in total bilirubin, alkaline phosphate, bile acids and liver enzymes. These results are common in many liver disease processes and diagnosis will be made by excluding other conditions.

Signs and symptoms

Obstetric cholestasis usually presents after the 30th week of pregnancy. Typically, the woman complains of pruritus in the palms of the hands and the soles of the feet in the absence of a rash. As pregnancy progresses, pruritus spreads from these areas to the trunk and the face. The sensation is severe and distracting and prevents adequate sleep as it is more noticeable at night. The women will appear tired and irritable, with no obvious signs apart from excoriation of the skin from scratching.

A total of 50% of women will go on to develop mild jaundice occasionally with symptoms of fever, abdominal discomfort and nausea and vomiting (Crafter 2003). These women may notice that their urine is darker and their stools paler than usual.

Treatment

The objective of treatment is to relieve maternal symptoms while improving fetal outcome. Ursodeoxycholic acid 10 mg/kg per day improves symptoms and biochemistry without any reported adverse effects on the fetus (Elias 2002). Topical treatments have limited effect, as does use of an antihistamine. Whatever treatment is used, vitamin K is also required as cholestasis reduces the absorption of fat soluble vitamins leading to vitamin K deficiency.

The woman with obstetric cholestasis may find a modification of diet to one that is low in fats reduces the severity of pruritus. An increase in fluid intake will also assist in the excretion of toxins from the body. Reducing stress is useful, as many women have recognized that the itchiness increases in high stress situations (Nichols 2005). External irritation can be reduced by moisturizing the skin, taking cool baths and wearing loose clothing.

Postnatally, the symptoms of pruritus should resolve quickly. However, some women continue to experience itching for up to 8 weeks postpartum. These women should be closely monitored to ensure the condition does disappear, as the continued presence of pruritus may indicate another underlying disease process (RCOG 2006).

Prognosis

The fetus is at increased risk of pre-term labour, fetal distress and stillbirth but elective delivery at 37–38 weeks avoids these in most cases. However, predicting fetal distress and demise is difficult in obstetric cholestasis with fetal monitoring proving normal only hours before death. The cause of fetal death is thought to be due to the increased levels of bile acids in the fetal circulation providing an environment incompatible with life. This condition carries a fetal mortality rate of up to 11–20% in untreated cases (Mullally & Hansen 2002).

For the woman, there is an increased risk of postpartum haemorrhage due to dysfunction of the liver and thus the production of coagulation factors. The incidence of gallstones is also increased.

The neonate

Due to the reduced production of vitamin K in the mother, the neonate should be given intramuscular vitamin K soon after birth to prevent haemorrhagic disease.

Future pregnancies

Obstetric cholestasis recurs in 40–60% of future pregnancies. Care must also be taken with the use of oestrogens in the contraceptive pill or during hormone replacement therapy (Coombes 2000).

RELATED DISORDERS

Gallstones

Gallstones are crystalline bodies formed in the gallbladder from the normal or abnormal constituents of bile. Cholesterol stones are the most common but calcium and bilirubin can also be the main constituent. Cholesterol stones are formed when there is too high a proportion of this substance in bile compared with bile salts, due to a combination of factors such as a familial tendency and body weight. Cholesterol production is increased in pregnancy and this and the associated decrease in muscle tone of the gallbladder results in an increased risk of developing stones. Acute cholecystitis is however, rare.

Many affected people are symptomless. Others will experience a range of symptoms from mild indigestion following ingestion of fat to severe debilitating biliary colic. The presence of gallstones may lead to inflammation of the gallbladder, cholecystitis, or stasis of bile – cholestasis, which can lead to dysfunction of the liver. Small stones tend to cause more acute problems as they may escape into the ducts.

Treatment is to surgically remove the stones by cholecystectomy, although this is avoided during pregnancy as far as possible.

Cholecystitis causes pain and tenderness in the right upper abdominal quadrant or mid-epigastrium. Fever, nausea and vomiting and leucocytosis (increased white blood cell count) are signs and symptoms of this condition. Jaundice may develop if the inflammation involves the biliary ducts (Box 12.2). Treatment is by rest, intravenous fluids, analgesics and antibiotics.

Acute fatty liver

Acute fatty liver is a rare disorder that usually appears during the third trimester and is commonly associated with pregnancy induced hypertension (Blackburn 2002). An incidence of between 1 in 7000 and 15000 has been recorded (Mjahed et al 2006). The condition, which has an unknown cause, is associated with a high maternal and fetal morbidity and mortality rate. Maternal mortality has been recorded as up to 18%, and is related more to complications than the disease itself (Ko & Yoshida 2006). Fetal mortality is associated with the need for a pre-term birth and may be as high as 20% (Tein 2000).

Typically, this condition is associated with obesity and the patient will present in the third trimester with headache and vomiting. Her condition will rapidly deteriorate with severe abdominal pain, jaundice and drowsiness. She may also show signs of renal failure and hypoglycaemia.

On examination, the woman may have a normal sized but tender liver, but on ultrasound examination the liver will show fat infiltration. Liver enzymes will be moderately raised. Treatment will involve correction of any coagulopathy with fresh frozen plasma and immediate delivery. Recovery is usually good but a recurrence of up to 25% has been noted (Tein 2000).

Viral hepatitis

Viral hepatitis is the most common cause of jaundice in pregnancy. Hepatitis is inflammation of the liver and although the condition shows similar signs and symptoms, treatment and prognosis depend on the cause. Symptoms include malaise, joint pain, abdominal pain, diarrhoea and vomiting, fever, hepatomegaly and jaundice. Viral hepatitis may be caused by:

Hepatitis A

Caught through contaminated food or water but this rarely occurs in developed countries.

Hepatitis B

Caught through sexual contact, intravenous drug use and blood contact or transfusion. A vaccination is available to prevent infection.

Hepatitis C

Transmitted through blood and carries a high mortality rate.

Other causes of hepatitis

Other causes of hepatitis are alcohol abuse, drug therapy, metabolic disorders and toxins. Viral hepatitis occurs in 1 in 1000 pregnancies (Crafter 2003) and is commonly caused by the hepatitis B virus. Hepatitis B infection is showing an alarming rise in the UK and is all the more serious because many infected individuals are asymptomatic or have symptoms that mimic influenza (Evans 2006). This virus can be transmitted across the placenta and the infant will be at increased risk of liver dysfunction in later life.

Diagnosis is made based on the woman's lifestyle and history. Treatment will be based on symptoms and infection control measures instituted where necessary.

REFERENCES

Alstead E M, Nelson-Piercy C 2003 Inflammatory bowel disease in pregnancy. Gut 52:159–161

Blackburn S 2002 Maternal, fetal and neonatal physiology: A clinical perspective, 2nd edn. WB Saunders, Philadelphia

Bruno M 2004 Irritable bowel syndrome and inflammatory bowel disease in pregnancy. Journal of Perinatal & Neonatal Nursing 18(4):131–135

Bush M C, Patel S, Lapinski R H, Stone J L 2004 Perinatal outcomes in inflammatory bowel disease. Journal of Maternal, Fetal and Neonatal Medicine 15(4):237–241

Coombes J 2000 Cholestasis in pregnancy: A challenging disorder. British Journal of Midwifery 8(9):565–570

Crafter H 2003 Problems of pregnancy. In: Fraser D M, Cooper M A (eds) Myles textbook for midwives, 14th edn. Churchill Livingstone, Edinburgh, p 309–310

Elias E 2002 Liver disease in pregnancy. Medicine 30(12):51–52

Evans N 2006 Hepatitis B. Practice Nursing 17(5):248–253

Kenyon A P, Girling J, Nelson-Piercy C et al 2002 Pruritus in pregnancy and the identification of obstetric cholestasis risk; a prospective prevalence study of 6531 women. Journal of Obstetrics and Gynecology 22(Suppl 2):515–519

Ko H H, Yoshida E M 2006 Acute fatty liver of pregnancy. Canadian Journal of Gastroenterology 20(1):25–30

Langarragard V, Pedersen L, Gislum M, Norgard B Sorensen H T 2007 Birth outcome in women treated with azathioprine or mercaptopurine during pregnancy: a Danish nationwide cohort study. Alimentary Pharmacology and Therapeutics 25(1):73–81

Mjahed K, Charra B, Hamoudi D, Noun M, Barrou L 2006 Acute fatty liver of pregnancy. Archives of Gynecology and Obstetrics 274(6):349–353

Mullally B, Hansen W 2002 Intrahepatic cholestasis of pregnancy: a review of the literature. Obstetrical and Gynecological Survey 57:47–52

Murray I 2003 Change and adaptation in pregnancy. In: Fraser D M, Cooper M A (eds) Myles textbook for midwives. Churchill Livingstone, Edinburgh, p 321–355

Nichols A 2005 Cholestasis of pregnancy: a review of the evidence. Journal of Perinatal & Neonatal Nursing 19(3):217–227

Riely C A, Fallon H J 1999 Liver diseases. In: Burrow G N, Duffy T P (eds) Medical complications during pregnancy, 5th edn. WB Saunders, Philadelphia

Royal College of Obstetricians and Gynaecologists 2006 Obstetric cholestasis. Guideline 43. RCOG, London

Somani R A 2003 Appendicitis in pregnancy: a rare presentation. Canadian Medical Association Journal 168(8):1020

Tein I 2000 Metabolic disease in the fetus predisposes to maternal hepatic complications of pregnancy. Pediatric Research 47(1):43–45

Index